Intravenous Therapy

Teresa M.D. Finlay
RGN, OncNC, BSc (Hons), MSc, Cert THE.
Senior Lecturer
Oxford Brookes University
Oxford
UK

Blackwell
Science

© 2004 by Blackwell Science Ltd
a Blackwell Publishing company

Editorial offices:
Blackwell Science Ltd,
9600 Garsington Road, Oxford
OX4 2DQ, UK
    Tel: +44 (0) 1865 776868
Blackwell Publishing Inc., 350 Main
Street, Malden, MA 02148-5020, USA
    Tel: +1 781 388 8250
Blackwell Science Asia Pty Ltd,
550 Swanston Street, Carlton,
Victoria 3053, Australia
    Tel: +61 (0)3 8359 1011

The right of the Author to be
identified as the Author of this Work
has been asserted in accordance with
the Copyright, Designs and Patents
Act 1988.

First published 2004

Library of Congress Cataloging-in-
Publication Data
Finlay, Teresa (Teresa M.D.)
    Intravenous therapy / Teresa M.D.
Finlay. – 1st ed.
        p.   ;   cm. – (Essential clinical
skills for nurses)
Includes bibliographical references
and index.
        ISBN 0-632-06451-X (pbk. : alk.
paper)
        1. Intravenous therapy.
        2. Injections, Intravenous.
        3. Nursing.
        [DNLM: 1. Injections,
Intravenous–nursing. WB 354 F511i
2003]   I. Title.   II. Series.

RM170.F56 2003
615′.6–dc21
                                2003012134

ISBN 0-632-06451-X

A catalogue record for this title is
available from the British Library

Set in 9 on 12pt Palatino
by SNP Best-set Typesetter Ltd.,
Hong Kong
Printed and bound in Great Britain
using acid-free paper
by TJ International Ltd, Padstow,
Cornwall

For further information on Blackwell
Publishing, visit our website:
www.blackwellpublishing.com

Contents

Foreword

Health care has benefited from a lengthy relationship with intravenous therapy throughout recent centuries. In fact, intravenous therapy continues to play a central role in the delivery of many modern day investigations and treatments. Therefore, it is of no surprise that this book has been written, but readers may ponder on the timing of such a publication. The answer is simple; in the world of intravenous therapy we are at a point of tumultuous transition. A period of development and change that can only strengthen the nursing contribution to intravenous therapy.

It is only in recent years that we have seen an increase in the nursing contribution to intravenous therapy. These changes have coincided with an abundance of national initiatives such as the scope of professional practice, the publication of numerous national guidelines related to intravenous therapy, including blood transfusion and central venous catheter care, and the development of vascular access teams. Developments over the last two decades have seen skills associated with intravenous therapy being merged with the long list of essential skills for registered nurses. Whether the issues are geographical, professional or skills-based, intravenous therapy holds no boundaries. Teresa Finlay has brought this philosophy together into one easy-to-read text. It may be presented as a beginner's guide, but the combination of practicality and essential information should ensure a place for this text on any practitioner's bookshelf.

In my daily practice I meet nurses who are often faced with the riddles and complexities of intravenous therapy. This essential guide will be an invaluable resource.

Teresa begins her book with an overview of role expansion, answering those often asked questions related to certification, moving between organisations and supervised practice, to name but a few.

Chapter 2 clearly integrates related anatomy and physiology, access devices and their potential effect upon the body, demonstrating how the integrity of normal structures can be disrupted during intravenous therapy. The most compelling component of Chapter 3 is the philosophy that demonstrates that even if you have not inserted a vascular access device or you are not administering intravenous medication, you still need to be aware of the device and how your patient should be cared for with such a device in place. Together, Chapters 4, 5 and 6 deliver an impressive practical guide that ranges from the reconstitution of medication, through the topics of fluid balance, blood component therapy and parenteral nutrition. It concludes with an essential guide to pharmacology and drug calculations.

Working within a specialised area of practice such as infusion therapy, I am often fearful that intravenous care may degenerate into nothing more than a collection of tasks. Within this guide, Teresa has encompassed the range and diversity of skills and knowledge required as a foundation for the delivery of safe, integrated, corroborated, effective and reliable patient-centred intravenous care.

Andrew Jackson
Consultant Nurse
Intravenous Therapy & Care,
Rotherham General Hospital NHS Trust, UK

Preface

Intravenous (IV) therapy is becoming ubiquitous in health care, impacting on nurses, midwives and many other health care professionals' daily practice. The administration of infusions or drugs and the care of venous access devices are routine aspects of patient care. It is not acceptable that patients should suffer avoidable injures from thrombophlebitis, infiltration or extravasation, and standards of practice are subject to scrutiny and are increasingly being questioned by patients. To this end it is clear that all practitioners involved in caring for patients with IV access and receiving IV therapy should have the knowledge and skills to enable them to deliver the highest standards of care to their patients.

Currently there is no national standard for IV therapy practice or education. Policy and training are locally agreed and delivered with variation nationally. Since the advent of clinical governance and evidence-based practice this is no longer satisfactory, and a nationally recognised programme of education needs to be adopted. The Royal College of Nursing (RCN) Intravenous Therapy Forum is working to develop a national standard based on guidelines developed by the Infusion Nurses Society in the United States of America. In addition, the emergence of expert practice and nurse consultant roles in practice areas directly relating to IV therapy is driving the change and development in IV therapy practice nationally.

The principles covered by this book aim to fulfil the RCN IV Therapy Forum standards and provide an essential grounding for good practice to support practitioners' knowledge development prior to gaining or updating practical experience and competence. The first chapter of the book covers issues relating to competence and practising with accountability. In the light of the rising numbers of errors in drug administration and increasing litigation, the importance of understanding legal and professional issues cannot be underestimated. Fluid and electrolyte balance and circulatory anatomy and physiology inform decision-making in IV therapy and are addressed in Chapter 2, drawing on examples directly associated with IV therapy practice. In addition, the implications of different types of IV access are introduced. Chapter 3 considers the devices which are used to gain IV access, their characteristics, uses and the care of patients having a device inserted, or with one in place. Practical, step-wise information about administering drugs and infusions is covered in Chapter 4 with examples of common practice situations and how to approach them. Chapter 5 covers infusion fluid therapy including blood and blood product transfusion, with information on different fluid types, when they are used and how they should be stored and administered. This includes parenteral nutrition though it is clear that this text is not comprehensive, and additional resources should be sought to develop skills in this area. Finally, the pharmacological aspects of IV therapy are considered in Chapter 6. General information about pharmacokinetics and pharmacodynamics precedes material about the effects of different methods and timing of administering IV therapy and details of resources for information about drugs and their administration. Calculation formulae are described with examples of calculations commonly undertaken in practice and there are test questions with answers for practice. Each chapter directs the reader to its contents, with clear summary points to conclude. In addition, useful resources for information are listed at the end of each chapter to enable further exploration of the topic as desired.

In aiming to provide a textbook covering all the fundamental aspects of knowledge required for IV therapy practice, the book does not seek to provide comprehensive information on all areas related to the subject. It is anticipated that readers are learning or refreshing their knowledge about the fundamental aspects of IV therapy before going on to build on or adapt them to their specialist areas of practice. For this reason the book does not cover cytotoxic chemotherapy administration, specialist issues related to paediatric IV therapy, community IV therapy or venepuncture and cannulation. There are other texts that cover these issues comprehensively and within the framework of more specialist knowledge specific to that area of practice.

The use of the term health care professional in the text refers to any qualified, registered practitioner in health care. The abbreviation IV is used to mean either intravenous or intravenously depending on the context. All the scenarios detailed in the text are fictitious and do not intentionally bear any resemblance to actual people or events.

It is hoped that this book will be adopted to provide new health care professionals with a good fundamental knowledge of the principles of IV therapy from which to develop safe, evidence-based practice for their patients.

Teresa Finlay
Oxford 2003

Acknowledgements

I would like to express my thanks to the following people for their inspiration, help and support in the development of this book:

- the patients;
- the intravenous therapy team at the Royal Marsden Hospital, and Val Speechley, who collectively awakened my interest in IV therapy practice;
- the teams with whom I have developed and delivered IV therapy distance learning materials and study days; the Nightingale Institute at King's College London, particularly Tina Day, the Practice Development Team and Kate Gee at University Hospitals Birmingham and the IV therapy working group at the Oxford Radcliffe Hospital Trust;
- Helen Hamilton, the Line Insertion and TPN teams at the Oxford Radcliffe Hospital Trust;
- Jill Kayley, Community IV Therapy Specialist Nurse;
- Sarah Blackburn, pharmacist;
- James Walthall;
- my colleagues and students;
- my family and friends;
- my partner Bob.

I would like to dedicate the book to my grandparents George and Isa Jervie, who were pharmacists; my grandmother has taken a keen interest in the progress of the project despite the major changes in practice since my grandparents' dispensing days.

Expanding Practice in IV Therapy

1

INTRODUCTION

With broadening responsibilities in health care and the recognised need for evidence-based practice, practitioners must have a working understanding of the professional and legal implications of their actions in advance of developing their practice. This is true for those involved in giving patients IV therapy, particularly as this aspect of care is potentially highly dangerous, but is becoming more relevant to almost all areas of practice. This chapter considers:

❏ competence; how to gain, develop and maintain competence in IV therapy;
❏ accountability; the issues of authority and autonomy and the legal implications of practising with accountability;
❏ evidence-based practice (EBP); the need for knowledge and the relationship of EBP to accountability.

COMPETENCE

Health care professionals (HCPs) involved in IV therapy have a duty to provide a reliable, safe standard of care to patients in a competent, skilled manner. In order to do so there are several steps to take to achieve competence (see Fig. 1.1).

Knowledge

It is essential that practitioners first develop (or update) a firm knowledge of:

- accountability;
- circulatory anatomy and physiology;

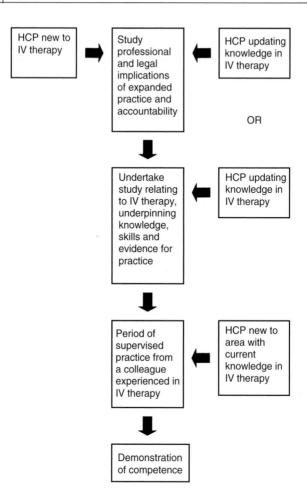

Fig. 1.1 Pathway to achieving or demonstrating competence in IV therapy administration

- fluid and electrolyte balance;
- techniques and equipment for IV therapy administration;
- pharmacology;
- administration of fluids, blood and blood products;
- risk management specifically relating to IV therapy;
- the possible effects of treatment on the patient, physically, socially and psychologically.

Knowledge is usually gained partly from studying these principles using learning packs or attending study sessions or a combination of both. Additionally, understanding of these principles is gained and reinforced by working with experienced colleagues.

Certificates

Having completed a period of study, most health care professionals are pleased to receive a certificate. The certificate constitutes evidence of attendance on the programme of study, and should be kept in the practitioner's portfolio. It is important to realise that this is no demonstration of ability. The practitioner's skill lies in their ability to apply the knowledge gained to practise and develop their competence in IV therapy.

Developing competence

Supervised practice

Having gained knowledge in the aspects detailed above, novice health care professionals should practise administering IV therapy in their clinical area with the supervision of a competent, more experienced colleague. This person is usually identified by the senior practitioner or the manager responsible for practice in that clinical area. The period of supervision is likely to vary from one practitioner to another. The aim is for the novice practitioner to develop competence in IV therapy with the guidance, facilitation and support of their supervisor.

Assessment

After a period of supervised practice both the novice and the supervisor should agree that the practitioner has demonstrated competence in administering drugs intravenously in their area of clinical practice. It is recommended that this is not assessed on a single occasion but over a period of time. 'One-off' assessments do not necessarily indicate competence. Drivers with valid driving licences gained at a single driving test do not necessarily drive safely! They did so only at the time of the test. Practitioners experienced in IV therapy, coming to a new clinical area may require a minimal period of supervision before it is agreed that they are competent to practise independently.

An example of clinical competences suitable for IV therapy is in Box 1.1 and such a form may be signed by both the practitioner and their supervisor. This form (copied to the manager for their records) will be retained by the practitioner for their

---

Box 1.1 Competences for IV drug administration

Elements of competence	Date and signature	
	Nurse	**Supervisor**
(1) Describes the rationale for administering drugs intravenously		
(2) Describes circumstances where it would be inappropriate to administer a drug intravenously, and alternative action to take		
(3) Describes the risks associated with intravenous drug administration		
(4) Demonstrates knowledge of the drugs routinely administered intravenously in that clinical area		
(5) Describes and/or diagnoses the signs and symptoms patients exhibit if a drug reaction occurs		

Elements of competence	Date and signature	
	Nurse	**Supervisor**
(6) Describes and/or takes the appropriate action in the event of a patient experiencing a drug reaction		
(7) Correctly calculates the doses, volumes and rates of drugs to be administered intravenously		
(8) Demonstrates appropriate techniques and actions in preparing drugs for administration intravenously		
(9) Demonstrates safe practice in the administration of prescribed intravenous medication		
(10) Demonstrates appropriate techniques in the administration of intravenous drugs as: • bolus injections • infusions over time		
(11) Demonstrates health-promoting practice in caring for patients' intravenous access and administering drugs to patients		
(12) Describes how to act appropriately in the event of a drug error or adverse incident associated with administration of intravenous drugs		
(13) Demonstrates awareness of their professional accountability		
(14) Demonstrates knowledge of available resources relating to drug information, local policy and current evidence for practice		

professional portfolio, along with any completed learning packs and information from the study sessions relating to IV therapy, and a certificate of attendance. Together these items provide *evidence* of the practitioner's development, though it is important to remember that though they support demonstration of competence, they do not prove it.

Updating knowledge and competence

Practitioners are responsible for keeping their knowledge and skills updated and may (as shown in Fig. 1.1) repeat study sessions about the legal and professional aspects of practice and IV therapy, or just those relating to IV therapy, depending on their needs and the provision of training available.

Moving to a different Trust

It has been the case that practitioners competent in IV therapy have been required to complete the whole process of study, supervision and assessment of competence when moving to a new Trust or health care institution. This is wasteful of time and resources, as well as indicating a lack of understanding and respect for professional practice. Whilst local policy should be followed for reasons of vicarious liability, practitioners who have evidence to support their practice should only have to demonstrate their knowledge and competence in order to give IV therapy. If, however, they have started working in a clinical environment unfamiliar to them, then there would be a case for undertaking specialised learning and a period of supervised practice in order to develop competence in giving different IV therapy to patients with different needs.

EXPANDED PRACTICE

Administering drugs to a patient intravenously has been considered to be an expanded practice role (for non-medical practitioners), or an additional area of practice for those who have not been taught these skills in their pre-registration course. This is despite the fact that approximately 80% of hospital patients receive some form of IV therapy, and an increasing number of patients in the community are treated with IV drugs or infusions (Dougherty 2000). The reason for this is that

IV drug administration was originally undertaken only by doctors. It is only in the last few decades that other health care professionals have started giving drugs IV. More recently some nursing pre-registration courses have included IV drug administration as part of the curriculum. For health care professionals who have not experienced this kind of education programme, IV therapy still constitutes an area of expanded practice, and expanding practice to undertake IV therapy should only be taken on by those who recognise this as beneficial to patient care, and for whom it is a requirement in their area of work.

For nurses, midwives and health visitors, expanded practice is supported by a code for practice laid down by their professional registering body – the Nursing and Midwifery Council (NMC) and stated in the Code of Professional Conduct (NMC 2002) (see Box 1.2). The expectation is that nurses keep

---

Box 1.2 The Code of Professional Conduct (NMC 2002)

- You must protect and support the health of individual patients
- You are answerable for your actions and omissions, regardless of advice or directions from another professional
- You have a duty of care to your patients, who are entitled to receive safe and competent care
- You must keep knowledge and skills up to date throughout your working life and take part regularly in learning activities that develop competence and performance
- You must possess the knowledge, skills and abilities required for lawful, safe and effective practice without direct supervision and acknowledge the limits of professional competence and only undertake practice and accept responsibilities for those activities in which you are competent
- If an aspect of practice is beyond your level of competence, you must obtain help and supervision from a competent practitioner until you and your employer consider that you have acquired the requisite knowledge and skill
- You have a responsibility to deliver care based on current evidence, best practice and, where applicable, validated research when it is available

---

patients' needs central to their decision-making, recognise their own level of competence and only take on aspects of practice for which they have current knowledge and skills and for which they can be accountable. There are similar expectations of practitioners in allied health professions (AHPs) as laid down in their respective codes of practice, and all are accountable for their practice.

ACCOUNTABILITY

Since the development of professional governing bodies such as the Nursing and Midwifery Council, the Radiographers Board and the Health Professions Council (for operating department practitioners and paramedics), health care professions have professionally and legally established practice that initiates and collaborates in patient care rather than merely following orders. In order to do this individual practitioners must be accountable for their practice. Essentially, accountability means being able to answer for actions taken or decisions made. Professionally this relates to the care given to patients in daily practice, whether giving IV drugs or any other aspect of care (Pennels 1997).

Authority and autonomy

To be accountable and to justify one's actions and decision-making, a health care professional must have the authority to act. Health care professionals automatically have this authority on registration as a qualified practitioner. This is on the basis of the education and training they received in order to gain registration. To be accountable, practitioners must also have autonomy. This means using one's judgement and acting on it so that practice can be defended or explained from the basis of knowledge rather than on the basis of tradition or myth. In other words, drawing up intravenous drugs as your colleague does 'because this is the way we do it here' is not acting autonomously. Drawing up the drugs in a safe manner based on available evidence and education is. Clearly, to practise with accountability, practitioners' knowledge must be maintained and updated. One cannot rely on what one learnt several years ago as the current knowledge for best practice. Neither inexperience nor ignorance of current practice in health care or the professional or legal issues involved in health care is an excuse for poor care or causing harm to a patient (Glover 1999). As can be seen from the development of accountable professions, carrying out orders from another professional is also no protection from liability if that causes harm to a patient (Dimond 2002) (see Box 1.3).

Legal aspects of accountability

Health care professionals are accountable in four areas in law (Dimond 2002). If a patient suffers any harm whilst receiving health care, then depending on the severity of the incident the professionals involved may be called to account in one or all of these areas (Table 1.1).

(1) Accountability to the patient enables patients to trust the professionals caring for them and expect the professionals to practise accountably. A patient or their relatives may

---

Box 1.3 To take orders?

A staff nurse new to the ward is given a prescription for a patient by the Senior House Officer. This is for a large, intravenous dose of a drug with which she is unfamiliar. She tells the SHO she will need to query it with the on-call pharmacist and that she is unprepared to give the drug as prescribed. The SHO is angry and decides to give the drug herself. After the SHO has left the ward, the patient becomes gravely ill and subsequently dies.

If the nurse had given the drug, both she and the SHO would be liable for negligence. This would be because the SHO had prescribed it, and the nurse had given a drug she was not familiar with because she was ordered to. In refusing to give the drug the nurse was practising accountably and within the law.

Table 1.1 Areas of legal accountability (Dimond 2002)

Area	Aspect of law	Where cases are heard
(1) Patient	Civil law	Civil court
(2) Professional	Professional body's code of practice	Professional hearing by professional body
(3) Public	Civil or criminal law	Criminal court
(4) Employer	Contract of employment, employment law	Employment tribunal, disciplinary hearing in the workplace

have the right to sue the practitioner for negligence in the civil courts in the event of the patient suffering harm.

For negligence to occur three conditions must apply:

- the professional must owe the patient a duty of care;
- the duty of care must be breached;
- the patient must suffer harm as a result.

All registered professionals automatically owe patients a duty of care by means of their registration. For negligence to apply the professional must have acted in a manner that would not be supported by their professional body, that would breach their duty of care, and cause the patient harm (Dimond 2002). In the fictional example in Box 1.4 the staff nurse had breached his duty of care by incorrectly administering a drug infusion by the wrong (non-prescribed) route. Mr Ward's subsequent death clearly is the most extreme form of harm. Consequently Mr Ward's family would have a case for suing the staff nurse provided they could prove causation, because the people bringing the case are required to prove negligence. This could take the form of a personal action against the staff nurse in the civil court. Alternatively the family could sue the Trust employing the nurse (see Vicarious Liability below).

Box 1.4 A simple error?

Mr Ward was recovering from thoracic surgery. He had an epidural infusion of bupivacaine in situ and an intravenous patient-controlled analgesia infusion with morphine. The nurse caring for him was suitably qualified to administer IV and epidural drug infusions. When the infusions were complete the nurse changed infusion syringes, reconnecting them to the existing extension tubing, although these should also have been changed and clearly labelled. Half an hour after the infusions were changed, Mr Ward suffered a respiratory arrest, was admitted to ITU but died several days later. On investigation it transpired that a morphine infusion had been connected to the epidural catheter by the staff nurse in error.

---

(2) Professional liability means that in the example in Box 1.4 the incident is automatically reported to the NMC and a professional conduct hearing arranged. In this hearing, evidence about the staff nurse's action and any mitigating circumstances, including the nurse's conduct record, is taken into consideration. The committee decides, on the basis of the evidence given, whether the staff nurse should remain on the Register or not. The committee's responsibility is to decide whether or not the public needs to be protected from an incompetent practitioner, not to punish the nurse concerned. They are able to make recommendations about future supervision and education for the nurse concerned if it is decided that he is not to be struck off the Register. Those who are struck off the Register are not able to practise as a professional.

(3) Accountability to the public is concerned with action that constitutes a criminal and/or civil offence. Clearly, causing the death of a patient is a criminal offence, as in Mr Ward's case. In this event the coroner takes control of the case, orders a post-mortem and calls an inquest into the death. The police charge the staff nurse with an offence committed in connection with Mr Ward's death

(manslaughter, or murder if the staff nurse had the intent to kill) and prosecute the staff nurse in the Crown Court. It is the responsibility of the prosecuting barristers (acting on behalf of the public) to prove to the jury that the staff nurse is guilty of the offence beyond a reasonable doubt. If the jury's verdict is pronounced as guilty the sentence given is at the judge's discretion but follows the guidance laid down by the statute for issues of involuntary manslaughter (recklessness or gross negligence). Such cases are rare but usually attract a high media profile.

(4) Employers expect their employees to follow their reasonable instructions in the form of policies and procedures, using their professional skills and due care. If an employer (usually in the form of a manager and a personnel or human resources department in a Trust) feels that an employee has breached their contract of employment, then disciplinary action may be taken. The staff nurse caring for Mr Ward is immediately suspended from duty on full pay, pending an inquiry. The Trust could decide to dismiss the staff nurse regardless of the outcome of any other inquiry or court case. If he is struck off the Register by the NMC for the incident, the Trust could not continue to employ him – registration is a condition of employment for a staff nurse. If, however, he is not struck off the Register, the Trust could decide not to dismiss him but to demote him, move him to another department or put in place an expectation of completing a period of supervised practice and training and achieving an agreed set of outcomes or competences.

Vicarious liability

In addition to the staff nurse's accountability to his employer, the Trust has vicarious liability for its employees. This means that if employees practise within the guidelines stated by their employer, the Trust is held responsible for employees' actions. In the example in Box 1.4, the Trust Mr Ward was treated by is vicariously liable for the staff nurse's action but is unlikely to defend (contest) any case brought against them. Mr Ward's family might decide to sue the Trust rather than the staff nurse, and if so, it is likely that the Trust will settle for a sum of money in compensation to Mr Ward's family to avoid a court action which they are unlikely to win. On balance, suing the Trust is more likely to yield a resolution in the form of monetary compensation.

EVIDENCE-BASED PRACTICE

Practising with accountability means basing decisions in practice on sound, current knowledge. This is the same as evidence-based practice, a term which has become popular in health care, particularly in the last decade. To engage in evidence-based practice is to practise accountably rather than ritualistically, based on what is justifiable from the evidence, as opposed to what is merely 'done here'. Evidence-based practice has become fundamental to health care because it:

- improves the quality and effectiveness of care;
- will make the 'lottery' of treatments an obsolete approach;
- should increase confidence in health care and promote informed choices for patients;
- encourages the use of audit to monitor and improve health care;
- enables practitioners to practise accountably;
- provides value for money;
- will result in an improved body of knowledge on which to base practice (Sackett *et al.* 1996).

It is important to understand that evidence-based practice is not simply research-based practice. Evidence-based practice is a dynamic use of the sources listed in Table 1.2, which show that working in partnership with patients is an integral part of evidence-based practice (summarised in Fig. 1.2). This approach uses a health-promoting model for care and is important in IV therapy. For example, if a patient has experi-

Table 1.2 Sources of evidence

Evidence	Sources
Research	Literature, databases (being able to appraise the quality of research)
Theory	Literature
Practitioners' experiences	Reflection on practice
Patients and carers' experiences	Assessments, interviews, focus groups, literature, support groups
Experts and role models' practice and experience	Interviews, conferences, focus groups, literature
Policies and guidelines	Internet, local Trusts, Department of Health, specialist groups

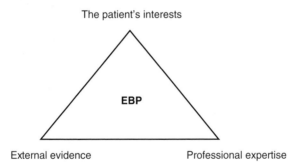

Fig. 1.2 Evidence-based practice

ence of giving their own IV therapy through a long-term central venous access device, they should continue to be involved in that aspect of care if hospitalised. If they become too ill to do so, their usual routine should continue to be acknowledged so that they could resume this part of their care in the future.

It is not always easy to put evidence-based practice into action. It requires a commitment to finding evidence and using it to change practice. This can involve a cultural shift within a team or an organisation to embrace change. Some people may find this threatening, actively obstruct change or lack the motivation needed. However, the knowledge and skills gained by health care practitioners expanding their practice and engaging in professional development, coupled with government and Health Service expectations for its implementation, are encouraging a shift towards evidence-based practice (Le May 2002).

Key points

- Novice practitioners need to develop a contemporary knowledge base
- Supervised practice is key to developing competence and confidence
- Competence should be assessed over time rather than on one occasion
- Practitioners need to maintain contemporary knowledge and skills
- Knowledge and skills are transferable
- Undertaking IV therapy administration requires an understanding of professional accountability and the law
- Accountability is not optional
- Accountability involves authority and autonomy in decision-making
- Practising accountably is a continuous process in which health care professionals monitor their professional performance as well as answer for the decisions they take in the course of their practice
- Evidence-based practice is fundamental to accountability

REFERENCES

Dimond, B. (2002) *Legal Aspects of Nursing* 3rd edn. Longman, Harlow.

Dougherty, L. (2000) Changing tack on therapy. *Nursing Standard*, **14**(30), 61.

Dowling, S., Martin, R., Skidmore, P. & Doyal, L. (1996) Nurses taking on junior doctors' work: a confusion of accountability. *British Medical Journal*, **312**(7040), 44–47.

Glover, D. (1999) *Accountability*. Nursing Times Clinical Monographs, Emap, London.

Lamb, J. (1999) Legal and professional aspects of intravenous therapy. In: L. Dougherty & J. Lamb eds, *Intravenous Therapy in Nursing Practice*. Churchill Livingstone, Edinburgh.

Le May, A. (2002) *Evidence-Based Practice*. Nursing Times Clinical Monographs, Emap, London.

NMC (2002) *The Code of Professional Conduct*. Nursing and Midwifery Council, London.

Pennels, C. (1997) Nursing and the law; clinical responsibility. *Professional Nurse*, **13**(3), 162–164.

Sackett, D.L., Rosenberg, W.M.C., Muir Gray, J.A., Haynes, R.B. & Richardson, W.S. (1996) Evidence-based medicine: what it is and what it isn't. *British Medical Journal*, **312**(7023), 71–72.

ADDITIONAL TEXTS

Muir Gray, J. (1997) *Evidence-based Healthcare: How to make Health Policy and Management Decisions*. Churchill Livingstone, Edinburgh.

Practitioners' own professional code or guidelines for practice

WEBSITES

Centre for Evidence-Based Medicine
http://cebm.jr2.ox.ac.uk

Centre for Evidence-Based Nursing
http://www.york.ac.uk/depts/hstd/centres/evidence

Cochrane Centre
http://www.cochrane.co.uk

Foundation of Nursing Studies
http://www.fons.org

NHS Centre for Reviews and Dissemination
http://www.york.ac.uk/inst/crd

Nursing and Midwifery Council
http://www.nmc-uk.org

Background Anatomy and Physiology and Venous Access

2

INTRODUCTION

To safely administer and manage patients' IV therapy, practitioners need an understanding of the physiology of fluid and electrolyte balance, dynamics and biochemistry as well as circulatory anatomy. The anatomical and physiological implications of using vascular access devices are significant and whilst these devices are becoming commonplace in health care, their risks should not be underestimated. This chapter will therefore examine:

❏ fluid and electrolytes; fluid compartments, electrolytes and movement between compartments;
❏ regulation of fluid and electrolyte balance;
❏ the circulatory system; vessels, blood flow and its dynamics;
❏ peripheral and central venous access; their indications and implications (detailed exploration of venous access devices is in Chapter 3).

FLUIDS AND ELECTROLYTES

In adults, body fluids are made up of water with solutes dissolved in it. Movement of both is a dynamic process, which maintains homeostasis in health. Disrupting this balance may seriously affect the individual's health in all the organs and systems of the body. Patients having intravenous therapy have direct access to the intravascular compartment, and disruption is potentially likely unless care is taken to prescribe and administer fluid and drugs appropriately.

Compartments

The water component of the body is greater than 50% (see Fig. 2.1). Its distribution is described as being in discrete compartments although there is always movement of water and electrolytes around the body and between the compartments. There are two main compartments:

- intracellular (fluid within individual cells);
- extracellular – further divided into:
  (1) interstitial fluid (between cells);
  (2) intravascular fluid or plasma.

Body fluid is made up of water with substances dissolved in it. These substances include:

- electrolytes;
- glucose;

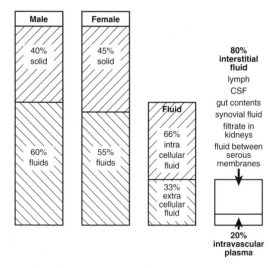

Fig. 2.1 Average body fluid distribution in adult males and females (from G.J. Tortora & S.R. Grabowski, *Principles of Anatomy and Physiology* 9th edn, John Wiley and Sons, New York, with permission)

- bilirubin;
- creatinine;
- urea.

Fluid balance is the presence and movement of the correct amount of water, electrolytes and other solutes between the compartments. Whilst there is always movement between compartments the net composition of each should always remain stable (see Table 2.1).

Factors which will vary fluid distribution and dynamics include:

- ageing: altered membrane structures inhibit fluid and electrolyte shifts;
- obesity and gender: more fat stored equates with less water volume;
- diet: a low protein diet or lack of electrolytes may affect levels and movement.

Imbalances occur when normal functions are disrupted and homeostasis is lost. Fluid and electrolyte imbalances occur as a result of:

Table 2.1 Composition of fluid compartments (Tortora & Grabowski 2000)

	Intracellular compartment	Extracellular compartment
Volume (average in litres)	25	16
Mainly composed of:	Water Glucose Amino acids Potassium Phosphate Magnesium Other electrolytes	Blood cells Antibodies Hormones Sodium Chloride Bicarbonate Calcium Other electrolytes

- increased intake and/or decreased excretion;
- decreased intake and/or increased excretion;
- acid–base imbalances, which are metabolic and may disrupt homeostatic regulation.

Electrolytes

Electrolytes are particles or ions which are electrically charged. Cations are positively charged, for example potassium, represented by K^+; anions are negatively charged, such as chloride, represented by Cl^-. Electrolytes are measured in the United Kingdom in millimoles per litre (mmol/l). They have four functions in the body.

(1) They control osmotic water movement between compartments. They tend to be confined to particular compartments depending on the electrolyte. Sodium is extracellular and potassium is intracellular, as demonstrated by their serum levels (see Table 2.2).
(2) They contribute to the maintenance of acid–base balance.
(3) The electrical charges they carry create action potentials for neurotransmission and control hormone and some neurotransmitter secretion.
(4) Some electrolytes are co-factors in the activity of enzymes.

Imbalances in electrolyte levels can have profound effects on homeostasis (see Table 2.2).

Movement

Fluids and electrolytes move between the compartments (Fig. 2.1) across semi-permeable membranes in such a way as to maintain balance. These movements occur according to a number of different processes.

(1) *Diffusion*: This is the movement of solutes down a concentration gradient, from an area of high concentration to an

Table 2.2 Summarised features of common electrolyte imbalances (Malster 1999, Tortora & Grabowski 2000)

Electrolyte	Low serum level Cause	Signs and symptoms	Treatment	High serum level Cause	Signs and symptoms	Treatment
Sodium 135–140 *mmol/l* Extracellular; maintains osmolality of extracellular fluid (ECF), essential for neuromuscular transmission.	• Vomiting • Diarrhoea • Excessive diuresis	• Muscle weakness • Dizziness • Headache • Confusion • Hypotension • Tachycardia • Shock	• Treat cause • Replace sodium and fluid losses and other electrolytes as needed • Reduce ECF fluid volume if indicated using diuretics and water restriction	• Excess intake • Dehydration • Renal failure	• Thirst • Fatigue • Restlessness • Hypertension • Oedema • Coma	Always maintain patient safety if confused. Monitor vital signs carefully until normal levels restored. • Treat cause • Rehydrate • Careful administration of hypotonic solutions with diuretics may be required • Low sodium diet may be indicated

Always maintain patient safety if confused. Monitor vital signs carefully until normal levels restored.

Table 2.2 *Continued*

Electrolyte	Low serum level Cause	Signs and symptoms	Treatment	High serum level Cause	Signs and symptoms	Treatment
Potassium 3.4–5.0 mmol/l; Intracellular; vital for neuromuscular transmission, intracellular function, cardiac muscle conductivity and acid–base balance.	• Vomiting • Diarrhoea • Excessive diuresis (use of diuretics) • Increased insulin level • Parenteral nutrition • Burns	• Cramps • Muscle weakness • Diminished reflexes • Increased diuresis • Nausea and vomiting due to paralytic ileus	• Treat cause • Replace potassium orally or IV	• Renal failure • Potassium replacement therapy • Low sodium level • Potassium sparing diuretics • Bowel obstruction	• ECG changes including ventricular ectopics leading to VF cardiac arrest • Anxiety, irritability • Fatigue • Nausea and vomiting	• Only administer hypertonic sodium chloride solution in extreme cases • Administer IV calcium to reduce depolarisation of membranes caused by raised potassium • Administer insulin and 50% glucose

	Causes	Signs and symptoms	Treatment	Causes	Signs and symptoms	Treatment
		• Cardiac dysrhythmias, flattened T waves		• Large volume blood transfusion • Chemotherapy due to cell lysis	• Diarrhoea	to shift potassium back into cells • Haemodialysis
Calcium 2.1–2.6 mmol/l Vital in neuromuscular transmission, cell wall structure, cardiac and skeletal muscle contraction and clotting. Also used for enzyme activation and hormone secretion.	• Inadequate intake • Lack of Vitamin D • Hypoparathyroidism • Hypoalbuminaemia • Pancreatitis • Large volume blood transfusion	• Finger tingling and numbness • Tetany • Hyperactive reflexes • Muscle cramps • Confusion • Seizures • Congestive cardiac failure	• Careful administration of calcium gluconate IV in short term • Treat cause	• Excessive intake • Excessive Vitamin D • Hyperparathyroidism • Renal tubule disease • Metastatic carcinoma involving bone	• Lethargy and weakness • Confusion • Depression • Nausea and vomiting • Increased diuresis • Renal stone formation • Calcification of soft tissues	• Treat the cause • Hydrate with 0.9% sodium chloride IV • Simultaneously use diuretics to promote calcium excretion • Monitor electrolyte levels closely

area of lower concentration, until equilibrium is reached, i.e. until solutes are evenly distributed in the solution. Carbon dioxide and oxygen move in this way.

(2) *Facilitated diffusion or transport*: This arises where molecules which are either large or highly electrically charged bind to transporters in the membrane. The transporters undergo a structural change when bound, and the molecule is released on the other side of the membrane. Though not strictly diffusion, this also happens where molecules move from areas of high concentration to those of lower concentration. Solutes which move in this way include glucose, urea and some vitamins.

(3) *Osmosis*: This occurs when water molecules move across plasma membranes from an area of high concentration of water to one of lower concentration of water. Alternatively it can be described as the movement of water across a plasma membrane from an area of low concentration of solutes to an area of high concentration of solutes to achieve equilibrium. The osmotic pressure exerted by one solution on another relates to tonicity. Usually the intracellular and extracellular tonicity are equal, so there is no overall (net) shift of water from one to the other. These two solutions are thus said to be *iso*tonic (*iso* – the same). Where a solution is *hyper*tonic (*hyper* – more than), water will move from the solution of lower tonicity to the hypertonic one; where a solution is *hypo*tonic (*hypo* – lower than), water will move from that solution to the one of higher tonicity.

For example, red blood cells are hypertonic to water, water is hypotonic to red blood cells. If red blood cells are placed in water, the water moves from the hypotonic area across the cells' membranes to the hypertonic area within the cells. Ultimately the cells will burst, as the intracellular tonicity is always higher than that of water. If the red cells were placed in 0.9% sodium chloride solution there would be no overall movement from one area to the other as the two areas are isotonic. However, if the red blood cells were put into a hypertonic solution such as 1.8% sodium chloride, water would move out of the cells (now hypotonic) and into the solution in an attempt to even the balance. The result would be that the cells would shrivel up. Thus most fluids infused intravenously are isotonic; this is why 0.9% sodium chloride solution is always used to flush intravenous cannulae or catheters and *never* water for injection.

(4) *Active transport*: There are substances which need to be actively moved across membranes in the opposite direction to their concentration gradient. Active transport uses energy from adenosine triphosphate (ATP) to transport molecules across membranes against the concentration gradient, the commonest example of this being the sodium/potassium pumps present in all cell membranes. This movement maintains the high levels of sodium in the extracellular compartments and the high levels of potassium inside cells. Other solutes actively transported across membranes include hydrogen, calcium and chloride, some amino acids and monosaccharides.

(5) *Filtration and reabsorption*: Bulk flow occurs passively as large molecules and the fluid they are in move together in response to pressure. Movement between capillaries and interstitial spaces occurs by bulk flow and is driven by blood hydrostatic pressure (BHP) and osmotic pressure. BHP is generated by the heart pumping and is higher at the arterial end of capillaries. In combination with the 'pull' of the osmotic pressure in the interstitial fluid, the 'push' exerted by the BHP results in filtration out of the capillary of fluids and solutes. BHP reduces through the capillary bed and at the venous end is sufficiently low that its 'push' effect is lower than the 'pull' effect of the blood osmotic pressure (even when combined with

the interstitial fluid osmotic pressure). The result is that fluids and solutes move back into the circulation at the venous end of capillary beds (Fig. 2.2) by reabsorption.

Regulation of fluids and electrolytes
Five of the body systems work together to regulate the fluid and electrolyte balance:

- gastrointestinal;
- renal;
- endocrine;
- cardiovascular;
- respiratory.

Gastrointestinal
Fluid and electrolyte movement is predominantly from the gut into the circulatory and lymphatic systems by passive and

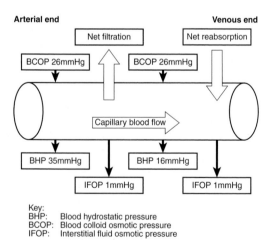

Fig. 2.2 Dynamics of fluid movement in capillaries (from G.J. Tortora & S.R. Grabowski, *Principles of Anatomy and Physiology* 9th edn, John Wiley and Sons, New York, with permission)

active transport. Large amounts of water, electrolytes and nutrients, both ingested and secreted into the gut, are absorbed mainly by the small intestine (see Table 2.3). The remaining water is absorbed from the colon, except for that excreted as part of faeces (approximately 100 ml every 24 hours).

Renal

Kidneys regulate the sodium and water content of the blood (and indirectly of the rest of the extracellular fluid). Changing sodium and potassium levels will affect the release of aldosterone and thus reabsorption of water and sodium (Fig. 2.3). Average urine production per day is dependent on intake and should be approximately 500 ml less than intake with a minimum of 30 ml/hour.

Endocrine

The relative 'concentration' of circulating blood – that is, how great an osmotic pressure it exerts, also called osmolality – is detected by receptors in the hypothalamus. If the blood osmolality is higher, the hypothalamus will increase its production of antidiuretic hormone (ADH). As a result, the kidneys will

Table 2.3 Electrolyte content and volume of gastrointestinal secretions (reproduced with permission from R.J. Eltringham & M.P. Shelley (1988) Rational fluid therapy during surgery. *British Journal of Hospital Medicine* **36**(9), 501–517)

Secretions	Volume (litres)	Sodium (mmol/l)	Potassium (mmol/l)	Chloride (mmol/l)
Saliva	0.5–1.5	20–80	10–20	20–40
Gastric	1.0–2.0	20–100	5–10	120–160
Bile	0.5–1.0	150–250	5–10	40–120
Pancreatic	1.0–2.0	120–250	5–10	10–60
Total volume	3.0–6.5			

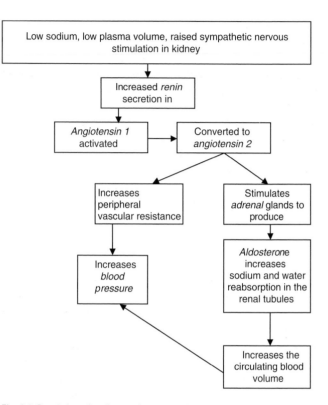

Fig. 2.3 Regulation of sodium and water uptake in the kidneys

reabsorb more water from the renal tubules, effectively 'diluting' the circulating blood. Less ADH is secreted if the blood osmolality is lower (it is more dilute) so that more water is excreted by the kidneys.

The thirst centre is also in the hypothalamus. A reduction in the intracellular fluid volume in these cells will stimulate thirst and thus increase fluid intake. As the fluid levels rise, the sensation of thirst diminishes.

Cardiovascular

The circulation of blood is vital to maintain tissue perfusion and thus the oxygenation, nutrition and excretion of cells in the body. Blood volume changes affect these processes and are carefully regulated by receptors in the cardiovascular system and the nervous system. If blood volume is sensed as being high by baroreceptors and stretch receptors in the aortic arch and carotid arteries, these receptors transmit signals to the sympathetic nervous system and vasodilation occurs. This ensures that the increased volume has a larger area to move in and pressure is not unduly raised. At the same time the raised blood volume leads to an increase in renal arterial pressure.

Glomerular filtration increases directly, with an increased urine production as the end result.

Respiratory

Respiration results in water loss, the volume lost being dependent on the environmental humidity (air water vapour content) and respiratory rate. The average water loss in expired water vapour is 400 ml in 24 hours.

Imbalance of fluid levels in any compartment will lead to disturbed electrolyte levels and affect acid–base balance and overall homeostasis. The implications of this depend on the degree of loss or gain. See Table 2.4 for the effects and management of fluid imbalance.

CIRCULATORY SYSTEM

A fundamental knowledge of the circulatory system is important to understand:

(1) how fluids are transported around the body and the cardiovascular system's role in fluid and electrolyte balance;
(2) vascular anatomy and the impact of intravenous therapy, cannulae and catheters on it.

The heart, vessels and blood collectively form the circulatory system. In order for blood to circulate around the entire

Table 2.4 Summary of fluid imbalances and management (Malster 1999)

	Causes	Signs and symptoms	Treatment
Hypovolaemia A decrease in the extracellular fluid volume due to lack of intake or excessive loss.	Severe fluid losses from the body: • vomiting • diarrhoea • diaphoresis (sweating) • haemorrhage or fluid movement into 'third' spaces: • bowel obstruction • ascites Decreased intake • starvation • shock • unconsciousness • mental illness	• Thirst • Decreasing diuresis • Reduced skin turgor • Tachycardia • Hypotension • Pale, clammy skin • Reduced consciousness • Increased urine specific gravity • Altered electrolyte levels depending on cause • Raised haematocrit in dehydration • Lowered haematocrit in haemorrhage (haematocrit = % blood volume made up of red blood cells)	• Replace fluid and electrolyte losses according to the cause • Manage replacement carefully to avoid overloading • Treat underlying cause • Aim to restore tissue perfusion Monitor vital signs including: • BP • Heart rate, peripheral pulses • Urine output • Central venous pressure if possible • Neurological state

Hypervolaemia			
An increase in the extracellular fluid due to excessive IV infusion (overload) or renal failure. Metabolic imbalances may precipitate overload.	• Excessive or rapid IV infusion • Infusion of hypertonic solutions IV • Renal failure • Liver failure • Cardiac failure leads to poor renal and liver perfusion resulting in fluid overload	• Increased diuresis • Oedema • Tachycardia • Hypertension • Raised JVP • Pulmonary oedema • Decreased urine specific gravity • Altered electrolyte levels depending on cause, low sodium • Raised haematocrit	• Reduce ECF volume using diuretics • Restrict water and sodium intake • Treat underlying cause • Dialysis if renal failure is the cause • Aim to restore normal volume Monitor vital signs including: • BP • Heart rate • Urine output • Respiratory rate, sounds • Oxygen saturation • Central venous pressure if possible

body and provide transportation of cells, water, electrolytes, nutrients and wastes, it is pumped by the heart first through the lungs for gas exchange and then through the rest of the body. Blood flows through the heart in one direction, each chamber being closed off from the next by valves.

The heart is a muscular organ with four chambers, lying just to the left of the midline of the thorax. Deoxygenated blood is pumped through the right side of the heart into the right atrium, and then from the right ventricle to the lungs, where carbon dioxide is released and oxygen binds to haemoglobin molecules in the red blood cells. On its return to the left side of the heart, oxygenated blood is pumped through the left atrium and ventricle and out to the aorta.

Blood vessels

From the aorta, blood is pumped through arteries and flows through capillaries, into veins and back to the right side of the heart. The blood vessels form a one-way system of transportation, arteries and veins sharing a common basic structure of three layers (Fig. 2.4).

(1) *Tunica externa* or *tunica adventitia* is the outer layer, which is made up of collagen, connective tissue and nerve fibres mainly of the sympathetic nervous system. This layer provides support, and the nerve impulses to it increase the tone of the vessel. More stimulation causes constriction whereas less results in relaxation. In veins this is the thickest of the three layers.

(2) *Tunica media* forms the middle layer. It is composed of smooth muscle fibres that run in rings around the vessel, and elastic fibres. Arteries have much thicker muscle layers than veins and have more flexibility to stretch or constrict in response to nerve impulses or pressure changes. Veins are more likely to collapse when pressure in the lumen is low, as the tunica media is much thinner. This layer is sen-

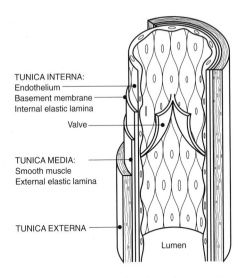

TUNICA INTERNA:
Endothelium
Basement membrane
Internal elastic lamina

Valve

TUNICA MEDIA:
Smooth muscle
External elastic lamina

TUNICA EXTERNA

Lumen

Fig. 2.4 Section through vein showing three-layered structure (from G.J. Tortora & S.R. Grabowski, *Principles of Anatomy and Physiology* 9th edn, John Wiley and Sons, New York, with permission)

sitive to changes in pH and temperature, chemical or mechanical irritation, which can result in spasm of the affected vessel. In arteries this may have serious consequences for the tissue distal to the artery, causing ischaemia and resulting in necrosis. This is why arteries are seldom cannulated and drugs almost never given directly into them.

(3) *Tunica intima* is the layer which lines the lumen of vessels. Adjacent to the tunica media is the basement membrane and innermost is the endothelium, a layer one cell thick, of squamous epithelial cells. It is the most fragile of the three layers and most prone to damage by the insertion of venous access devices. The intima is continuous through-

out the cardiovascular system and has particular properties to enable the smooth flow of blood around the system. It is also sensitive to pH, chemical and temperature changes. Valves in the venous system are made up of folds of endothelium in the walls of the veins which support the column of blood as it flows against gravity through the vein. Their presence prevents pooling of blood in the peripheral circulation, assisting its return to the heart.

Capillaries are fine vessels that connect arteries and veins and comprise only endothelium on their lumen and basement membrane surrounding the endothelium. Their function is to supply nutrients and remove wastes between blood and tissue cells via the interstitial fluid.

Blood flow

Blood pressure is the hydrostatic pressure exerted by the blood on the walls of a vessel. It is generated by contraction of the ventricles and large systemic arteries. Resistance to flow is caused by friction between blood and the vessel walls it is flowing past. The smaller the radius of a vessel the higher the resistance to blood flow and the greater the friction generated. Resistance is highest in arterioles and capillaries, whilst the large arteries and veins provide little resistance. The vasomotor centre in the brain and the sympathetic nervous system control contraction or relaxation of vessel walls. This changes vessel radius, and thereby alters resistance and blood pressure.

As blood flows from the heart, through the aorta and into progressively smaller vessels to the capillary beds, the pressure drops as it gets further from the heart. When it reaches the veins the drop in pressure continues until it is at 0 mmHg on entering the right ventricle. Venous return is dependent on several factors.

(1) A pressure of 0 mmHg in the right atrium facilitates venous return because it is lower than the pressure in the veins. If pressure in the right atrium is increased because of right-sided heart failure or diseased heart valves, for example, venous return is decreased and there is a build-up of blood in the venous circulation.

(2) The skeletal muscles in the legs and arms contract, pumping blood up the veins towards the heart. The pumping action simultaneously opens the valves in the veins. When the muscles relax, blood is prevented from flowing back down the veins due to gravity, because the valves open when the muscle relaxes stopping the down-wards flow of blood.

(3) Respiration induces pressure changes in the thorax. On inspiration the diaphragm contracts and increases the capacity of the thorax to allow the lungs to expand. This causes a decrease in intra-thoracic pressure but a simulta-neous rise in abdominal pressure. The higher pressure on the veins in the abdomen causes blood to move from the abdominal part of the veins to the thoracic part of the veins, including the inferior vena cava, where pressure is lower. On expiration, the pressures change but valves prevent blood flowing back down the veins.

Dynamics

Fluid flows from one point to another when the pressure is higher at the first point than at the distant one. In a tube, fluid should flow in a smooth, aerodynamic way – also known as 'laminar' flow, in which the fluid at the centre of the lumen flows more quickly than fluid at the edges. In blood vessels, laminar flow occurs and is slower at the edges owing to the resistance or friction between blood and endothelium. However, it all flows in the same direction. When fluid moves in a turbulent flow, though the overall movement is forward, the fluid flows in all directions (Fig. 2.5). This occurs when there is damage to the endothelium lining the vessel, or if the

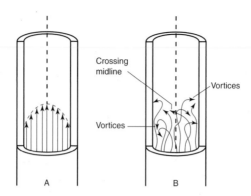

Fig. 2.5 Laminar and turbulent flow (from L. Dougherty & J. Lamb eds, *Intravenous Therapy in Nursing Practice.* Churchill Livingstone, Edinburgh, with permission)

lumen of the vessel changes abruptly, or if there is a very high flow through the vessel. Turbulent flow can sometimes be heard, such as through over-damaged heart valves which produce a 'heart murmur', or palpated such as through an arterio-venous fistula formed for haemodialysis. Where a venous access device (VAD) is present, or damage has been caused to a vein by the presence of one, flow will become turbulent, having previously been laminar, and will predispose the patient to development of a thrombus at the site of damage.

Damage to venous endothelium can be caused by mechanical or chemical means. Mechanical means include:

- using too big a cannula for the vein;
- poor technique inserting the cannula;
- a cannula which is inflexible and unable to bend with the vein as it moves;
- poor siting over a joint where flexion is frequent;

- poor fixing of the device allowing movement of the cannula in the vein.

Chemical means include:

- infection from the skin puncture wound on cannulation, or from contaminated infusions;
- fast infusions of large volumes of fluid into small veins;
- infusions of irritant solutions (due to pH, tonicity, chemical composition) (Scales 1999).

Initially, endothelial damage may simply be signified by mild tenderness over the vein concerned. This is due to irritation of the intima or endothelium and indicates phlebitis. This is a common but avoidable consequence of IV therapy arising where there is inflammation of one or more layers of the wall of a vein. When visible signs of inflammation are apparent, all three layers of the vein are inflamed, as well as the dermis and epidermis overlying it.

PERIPHERAL AND CENTRAL VENOUS ACCESS

In IV therapy the use of peripheral or central veins to achieve access is dependent on the principal reasons for the patient's therapy, the severity of their illness and the anticipated duration of the treatment.

Vascular access is required for:

- administration of fluids and drugs directly into the circulation;
- monitoring of central venous or arterial pressures or cardiac function;
- diagnostic procedures such as angiograms, in which the arterial blood flow through an organ or area of tissue is highlighted by the injection of radio-opaque contrast into the arterial supply to that area;
- treatment procedures such as angioplasty, where arterial supply may be modified to improve blood flow, or haemodialysis.

Peripheral venous access

The use of peripheral veins for IV access usually implies the use of the veins in the hand or forearm, though those in the feet or lower leg may be used. Peripheral venous access is intended for *short-term* therapy (hours or days). Each access site and device should be frequently monitored for signs of phlebitis, infection and infiltration or extravasation. The site must be changed at the earliest sign of complications and up to every 96 hours (Bregenzer *et al.* 1998, Laj 1998). The main reasons for using peripheral access include:

- fluid replacement;
- blood transfusion;
- drug administration.

The veins in the hands and forearms (lying reasonably superficially to the epidermis) are most commonly used due to the ease of access. Anatomically, risks of cannulating the forearm include the potential for arterial damage owing to the close proximity of veins to arteries. In addition, the considerable movement and flexure of the joints from fingers to elbow can cause discomfort at the cannulation site, damage the vein's intima, result in phlebitis and thus shorten the dwell time of the cannula (Dougherty 1999).

The site of peripheral cannulation in the forearms is determined by the anticipated use of the cannula. The larger the vein the greater the volume of blood that will flow through it in a given time.

The smaller veins in the dorsum of the hand should be used when it is possible to use a small device for administration of IV therapy for a short period (see Fig. 2.6), for example:

- patients receiving one-off IV injections such as sedation for endoscopy or minor general anaesthesia;
- short-term courses of intermittent injections of non-irritant drugs such as ampicillin or ranitidine;

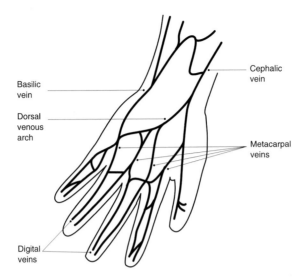

Fig. 2.6 Venous anatomy of the upper dorsum of the right hand (from L. Dougherty & J. Lamb eds, *Intravenous Therapy in Nursing Practice*. Churchill Livingstone, Edinburgh, with permission)

- small volume, short-term infusions of non-irritant drugs such as insulin for diabetics or opiates in patient-controlled analgesia infusions postoperatively;
- short-term, slow infusions of crystalloid fluid for maintaining hydration.

A larger vein should be used when a larger cannula is required or when higher blood flow is required for the treatment being administered, for example:

- Rapid infusion of fluid to rehydrate a patient or increase their blood volume. Rapid flow into a small vein will cause turbulence in the vein and damage the intima. In addition, fast flow will require a large cannula which should not be sited in a small vein (see below).

- Blood or blood product transfusion usually requires a larger diameter/gauge cannula to ensure the patency and flow through the cannula. Large-gauge cannulae will damage the intima of a smaller vein and so need to be inserted into a larger one.
- Infusion of a drug which may be irritant to the intima indicates administration into a larger vein with a more rapid blood flow to dilute the drug and minimise its effects on the delicate endothelium.
- If peripheral veins are collapsed due to shock, dehydration or hypothermia, a larger vein may be more easily accessed initially (Weinstein 2001).

Central venous access

Veins in the thoracic cavity, which drain directly into the right atrium, are classed as 'central' veins. The tips of central catheters lie either in the superior vena cava or in the right atrium of the heart. Access to central veins is by two means.

(1) A direct approach into the internal jugular vein or the subclavian vein is the most common route for central vein access (see Fig. 2.7). These routes are commonly used for short-term access, and often in emergency situations (see Table 2.5). Access may also be achieved via the femoral vein, though this is seldom used for patients outside critical care units (Scales 1999).

(2) An indirect route into a central vein (usually the subclavian in the first instance) is achieved with tunnelled and implanted central catheters (see Chapter 3, p 89). Peripherally inserted central catheters (PICCs) access the central venous system via the basilic, cephalic or median cubital veins in the arm (see Chapter 3, p 89). All these routes of access to the central venous system are used for longer-term IV therapy of weeks, months or even years in the case of tunnelled and implanted catheters (Gabriel 1999).

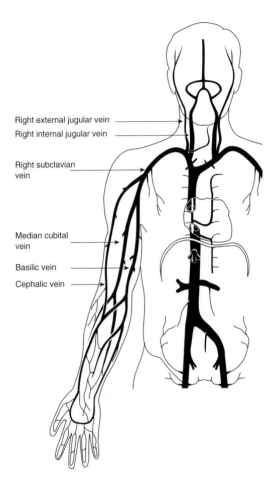

Right external jugular vein

Right internal jugular vein

Right subclavian vein

Median cubital vein

Basilic vein

Cephalic vein

Fig. 2.7 Venous anatomy of the upper body

Due to central veins' proximity to the heart and lungs, obtaining and maintaining central venous access is inherently dangerous. Both on insertion and in continuing care of patients with central venous access, steps must be taken to avoid, detect and act promptly when complications arise. The issues

Table 2.5 Indications for short- and long-term central venous access (Dougherty and Lamb 1999)

Short-term central venous access	Long-term central venous access
Monitoring central venous pressure	Administration of any long-term IV drug regimen • immunosuppressant drug therapy IV in transplanted patients • cytotoxic drug regimen for cancer patients • antibiotic regimen for patients with chronic infection or risk of same
Fast administration of fluids and/or blood to restore hydration and blood volume	Administration of parenteral nutrition
Administration of hyperosmolar solutions (includes parenteral nutrition)	Administration of fluids for hydration
Administration of vesicant cytotoxic drugs	Administration of blood products
Lack of peripheral venous access	Blood sampling

considered here relate to the effect on the patient of accessing central veins. Issues relating to the devices and their management will be examined in more detail in Chapter 3.

When inserting central venous access the main complications encountered include:

• *Pneumothorax*: Air enters the pleural space between pleura and lung on attempting to directly pierce the subclavian vein.

The patient will experience dyspnoea and may experience pain on inspiration and expiration. A pneumothorax should be confirmed or excluded with a chest X-ray (Weinstein 2001).

- *Haemothorax*: Blood leaks into the pleural space from damage to the subclavian vein or artery during the insertion procedure.

  The patient will experience the same symptoms as with pneumothorax with associated tachycardia and hypotension depending on the severity of haemorrhage into the pleura.

- *Arterial puncture*: This is usually clearly indicated by pusatile spurting of bright red blood due to puncture during the procedure and digital pressure should be applied until bleeding stops. However, there may be internal bleeding which is not immediately apparent. Haematoma formation with resulting tracheal compression and respiratory distress can result. Internal bleeding should be excluded with a chest X-ray (Weinstein 2001).

- *Atrial fibrillation*: The heart develops an atrial fibrillation (AF) rhythm in response to irritation from the tip of the device inserted when it rests in the right atrium against the wall of the heart.

  Patients experience tachycardia and possible hypotension, with the AF rhythm being evident on ECG (Gabriel 1999).

- *Air embolus*: Air may be entrained into the venous circulation during inspiration, reaching the pulmonary artery via the heart, during the insertion procedure of a direct central venous access device. It may also occur while the device is in situ around the catheter (less commonly), through an open-ended catheter, when an infusion is complete, or on removal of the device.

  Patients may experience dyspnoea, chest pain, reduced cardiac output, confusion, visual impairment and hemiparesis if this occurs. On insertion of devices patients should be laid flat or head down (in the Trendelenberg position) to prevent the action of gravity and reduce the likelihood of entraining air. This may also be adopted when devices are removed, or the patient may be asked to hold their breath after inspiration until an occlusive dressing can be applied (see Chapter 3, p 87) (Scales 1999).

- *Thrombosis*: On insertion of the device the central vein wall and intima will be damaged by the puncture wound. The site of damage and the presence of the catheter will cause platelets to adhere to the site of damage and the catheter. Large thrombi may form at the site or particles may break away and be carried to the pulmonary circulation, the myocardium and the brain by the circulation.

  Swelling of the area over, or distal to, the catheter insertion into the vein will cause patients discomfort; discolouration and coolness of the skin may become apparent. There may be difficulties in using the catheter for infusion or blood sampling. If emboli migrate to the lungs, heart or brain, symptoms of, respectively, severe dyspnoea, chest pain, and altered consciousness and hemiparesis may ensue (Wickham *et al.* 1992).

- *Infection*: This is a principal concern associated with venous access, and central venous access in particular. At all times, from preparation for insertion of a venous access device until after its removal, prevention of infection is of paramount importance, as the device provides access for micro-organisms to nutrient-rich blood and major organs, as well as for IV therapy. Within minutes of being placed, catheters are coated in fibrinogen and platelets that develop a 'fibrin sheath' around the device. This sheath helps bacteria to adhere to the catheter and shields them from antibiotics and natural immune defences (Weinstein 2001).

  The implications of infection for patients and their care will be explored in more detail in Chapter 4.

Intravenous therapy can adversely affect the structure of veins and the flow of blood through them. It can also restore fluid and haemodynamic balance, and quickly and effectively treat life-threatening conditions. Incorrectly managed, IV therapy can cause potentially lethal disruption to the body. Understanding the normal structure and function of the cardiovascular system, fluid and electrolyte balance and the potential means and effects of disruption should facilitate the prevention, or minimisation, of damage to a patient's vasculature and homeostasis when handling their IV therapy.

Key points

- Body fluid is water with solutes including electrolytes, glucose and proteins dissolved in it

- The body is 'divided' into three fluid compartments, although there is always movement of water and electrolytes between compartments

- Fluid balance results in a stable net composition of body fluids in each compartment, despite dynamic movement

- Electrolytes are charged atomic particles; the correct level of each is vital to control water movement, maintain acid-base balance, neurotransmission and enzyme activity

- Body fluids move between compartments by diffusion, facilitated diffusion, osmosis, active transport or filtration and reabsorption

- Five body systems combine to regulate fluid and electrolyte balance: gastrointestinal, renal, endocrine, cardiovascular and respiratory

- The circulatory system, comprising heart, vessels and blood, provides transport of cells, water, electrolytes, nutrients and wastes

- Blood vessels have a three-layer structure: tunica externa, tunica media and tunica intima, the latter being particularly fragile and prone to damage from VADs

- Blood usually flows in a smooth forward direction known as laminar flow

- Turbulent flow arises when there is vessel damage or a VAD is situated in a vein, and predisposes the patient to thrombus formation

- The use of peripheral or central veins to achieve venous access is dependent on the principal reasons for therapy, the severity of illness and the anticipated duration of therapy

REFERENCES

Bregenzer, T., Conen, D., Sackmann, P. & Widmenr, A.F. (1998) Is routine replacement of peripheral intravenous catheters necessary? *Archives of Internal Medicine*, **158**(2), 151–156.

Dougherty, L. (1999) Obtaining peripheral venous access. In: L. Dougherty & J. Lamb eds, *Intravenous Therapy in Nursing Practice*. Churchill Livingstone, Edinburgh.

Dougherty, L. & Lamb, J. eds (1999) *Intravenous Therapy in Nursing Practice*. Churchill Livingstone, Edinburgh.

Eltringham, R.J. & Shelley, M.P. (1988) Rational fluid therapy during surgery. *British Journal of Hospital Medicine* **36**(9), 501–517.

Gabriel, J. (1999) Long-term central venous access. In: L. Dougherty & J. Lamb eds, *Intravenous Therapy in Nursing Practice*. Churchill Livingstone, Edinburgh.

Laj, K.K. (1998) Safety of prolonging peripheral cannula and intravenous tubing use from 72 hours to 96 hours. *American Journal of Infection Control*, **26**(1), 66–70.

Malster, M. (1999) Fluid and electrolyte balance. In: L. Dougherty & J. Lamb eds, *Intravenous Therapy in Nursing Practice*. Churchill Livingstone, Edinburgh.

Scales, K. (1999) Vascular access in the acute care setting. In: L. Dougherty & J. Lamb eds, *Intravenous Therapy in Nursing Practice*. Churchill Livingstone, Edinburgh.

Tortora, G.J. & Grabowski, S.R. (2000) *Principles of Anatomy and Physiology* 9th edn. John Wiley and Sons, New York.

Weinstein, S.M. (2001) *Plumer's Principles and Practice of Intravenous Therapy* 7th edn. Lippincott, Philadelphia.

Wickham, R., Purl, S. & Welker, D. (1992) Long-term central venous catheters: issues for care. *Seminars in Oncology Nursing*, **2**(8), 133–147.

ADDITIONAL TEXT

Carroll, H. (2000) Fluid and electrolytes. In: M. Sheppard & M. Wright
eds, *Principles and Practice of High Dependency Nursing*. Baillière
Tindall/RCN, Edinburgh.

WEBSITES

Central venous access and monitoring
http://www.nda.ox.ac.uk/wfsa/html/u12/u1213_01.htm

Disorders of fluid and electrolyte balance
http://members.tripod.com/~lyser/ivfs.html

Anatomy and physiology
http://www.wiley.com/college/bio/tortora

Vascular Access Devices

3

INTRODUCTION

People with vascular access devices (VADs) in situ include almost all patients in acute care settings and some in continuing care or at home in the community. For the purposes of this chapter VADs refer to devices that provide venous access for the routine administration of drugs or fluids, monitoring of central venous pressure and withdrawal of blood samples.

Caring for patients' VADs is not difficult or time-consuming when incorporated into regular nursing care and drug administration, and it is vital to optimise their treatment. It is the responsibility of the nurse caring for the patient to care for *all* their needs, including managing their VADs, whether the nurse is giving drugs intravenously or not. If that nurse is in doubt or unsure of procedures involved, then advice and help must be sought and steps taken to gain the knowledge required to care for these patients appropriately. This chapter will show that neglecting this aspect of care may have significant or even disastrous consequences for patients. The chapter will examine:

- ❏ infection;
- ❏ peripheral venous access devices, their insertion, management and removal;
- ❏ midline catheters;
- ❏ central venous access devices, their risks, insertion, management and removal.

In order to optimise having a venous access device in situ, it is essential that patients' VADs are cared for observing fundamental standards, whatever the device being used (see Box 3.1).

> **Box 3.1** Fundamental standards for care of patients' VADs
> (adapted from Dolan & Dougherty 2000)
>
> Prevent infection
> Maintain a 'closed' system with as few connections as possible
> Keep the access 'patent' or free flowing
> Prevent damage to the device and associated equipment
> Minimise damage to the patient's vein

INFECTION

Whatever kind of intravenous access device is used, infection is a potential hazard to the patient from the time of insertion until after its removal. Insertion of the VAD through the skin into the bloodstream provides the route for organisms to enter the body and/or proliferate and set up an infection. Organisms involved in this may be either exogenous or endogenous, where *endogenous* ones are those which are already present on the patient's body and *exogenous* organisms are those which invade the body from elsewhere by cross-infection.

Causes of infection associated with IV therapy equipment can be divided into two groups: intrinsic and extrinsic contamination. *Intrinsic* contamination is caused in drugs, fluids or equipment prior to use for the patient's IV therapy, whilst *extrinsic* causes are attributable to contamination being introduced by the handling of drugs, equipment or the patient during the course of IV therapy (see Fig. 3.1).

Extrinsic contamination in IV therapy would lead to infection via the *extraluminal* route – the invading organisms would invade the patient's skin and travel down the outside of the device. This would usually result in the symptoms of infection within a week of insertion. Alternatively, with *intraluminal* colonisation, organisms spread from the interior of the fluid container, administration sets or injection bungs down the inside of the lumen of the device, and may be caused by either intrinsic or extrinsic contamination. Symptoms may only

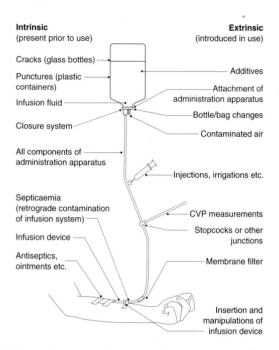

Intrinsic (present prior to use)

Cracks (glass bottles)

Punctures (plastic containers)

Infusion fluid

Closure system

All components of administration apparatus

Septicaemia (retrograde contamination of infusion system)

Infusion device

Antiseptics, ointments etc.

Extrinsic (introduced in use)

Additives

Attachment of administration apparatus

Bottle/bag changes

Contaminated air

Injections, irrigations etc.

CVP measurements

Stopcocks or other junctions

Membrane filter

Insertion and manipulations of infusion device

Fig. 3.1 Potential mechanisms for contamination of intravenous infusion systems (from L. Dougherty & J. Lamb eds, *Intravenous Therapy in Nursing Practice*, Churchill Livingstone, Edinburgh, with permission)

become apparent up to a month after insertion in central catheters.

Many patients with VADs are compromised immunologically and thus will be unable to 'fight' the infection effectively. These patients include those who:

- are poorly nourished;
- have an existing infection;
- are having antibiotic therapy;
- undergo numerous invasive procedures;

- are immunocompromised due to HIV or leukaemia;
- are immunosuppressed due to cancer therapy or anti-rejection transplant drugs;
- are elderly or under a year old.

All patients with VADs are at significantly higher risk of infection than those without, and strict observation of universal precautions and asepsis in all procedures is imperative to reduce this risk (Nystrom *et al.* 1983).

Preventing infection in IV therapy

Golden rules

The skin of either the patient, but more particularly health care workers, carry many of the organisms implicated in bacterial contamination associated with IV therapy, the most common being Staphylococci (Weinstein 2001). Health care personnel pose a significant threat because of their movement between patients, carrying infective organisms from one to another. This is particularly true when only a few nurses in a clinical area are able to administer drugs intravenously and they move from one patient to another, handling their IV therapy and VADs. The single most important and neglected factor in the prevention of cross-infection is *handwashing*. This must be undertaken thoroughly before and after every contact with a patient and their VAD, whether or not gloves are used (Philpott-Howard & Casewell 1994). *Asepsis* is mandatory whenever a VAD is inserted or removed, the site is exposed, or the system is 'broken' or disconnected for however short a time, in order to reduce the risk of extrinsic contamination. An effective strategy for improving practice in respect of infection associated with VADs is to involve patients in reminding staff about handwashing and cleaning devices before and after handling them. Patients should also be involved in monitoring their own devices and the exit site for signs of infection (Drewett 2000).

Insertion of the VAD

Cannulating a patient's vein, wherever the location of the insertion site or the procedure is undertaken, constitutes minor surgery and the principles of asepsis must be applied as with any surgical procedure. The preparation of the patient's skin prior to the insertion of the device is imperative to reduce the risk of colonisation of the insertion site, the device and the patient's blood with their skin flora. Chlorhexidine is thought to be a most effective skin cleansing agent (Maki *et al*. 1991) but for it to be effective the skin must be thoroughly rubbed for at least a minute and the solution then allowed to dry before the skin is punctured. Shaving should be avoided, as the abrasions caused by a razor will increase the likelihood of infection. Adequate skin cleansing at the site will include cleansing of any hair in the vicinity; it could be clipped with scissors prior to skin preparation if removal is thought to be really necessary.

Equipment and manipulation

Extrinsic contamination can be significantly reduced with the use of closed systems for administration and by reducing the frequency of manipulations of the system as much as possible. In addition, the use of effective handwashing, non-touch and aseptic techniques will minimise contamination (Hart 1999).

Infusion containers should be carefully examined against the light for leaks, cracks, particles or cloudiness before use, as these would indicate contamination of their contents and contraindicate their use. If contamination is suspected, the entire batch should be isolated from use and the manufacturer contacted. Fluid containers should not be hung for infusion for longer than 24 hours, as bacterial proliferation significantly increases after this time at room temperature (Weinstein 2001).

Sterile equipment packaging should be intact, sterilised and within the expiry date. *Administration sets* must be connected using non-touch techniques. The duration of use of administration sets needs to balance three issues:

- risks from manipulation;
- risks of contamination of the set if left in situ;
- the cost of equipment.

The less frequently the system is disconnected in order to change the administration set, the less likely complications associated with infection, embolism or haemorrhage are to occur. In particular, the less often the set is changed, the less manipulation will be implicated in causing contamination. However, if left connected to the patient's VAD, an administration set will show some contamination after 24 hours. This is minimal if the set is only used for the infusion of crystalloid fluids, and the benefit of a daily change of administration set is usually outweighed by the expense. Table 3.1 indicates when to change administration sets.

When adding drugs or fluids to containers or administration systems, asepsis must be observed both in drawing up the substance to be administered and when adding the drug or fluid. (Details of how to administer drugs are found in Chapter 4.) *Injection ports* reseal after repeated piercing with a 25G needle (orange), maintaining the 'closed' system. The reseal function will be damaged by repeated piercing with needles larger than 23G (blue). Before piercing an injection port it should be firmly rubbed with alcohol for at least a minute and the alcohol allowed to dry.

Three-way taps or stopcocks should only be used when absolutely necessary as they present a significant infection risk on several counts. The ports on three-way taps are open to contamination and swabbing is difficult as their surface is not flat; repeated turning of their mechanism and flushing with fluid enables contaminants to be easily infused into the patient's venous system.

By virtue of their function, three-way taps are frequently manipulated, thus significantly increasing the risk of contamination. Three-way taps should not be directly attached to a peripheral cannula (see Fig. 4.3). The manipulation of the tap

Table 3.1 Frequency for changing administration sets

Type of infusion set	Frequency of change	Rationale
Simple crystalloid infusion	72–96 hours	No significant increase in infection when left in situ up to 96 hours (Laj 1998).
Crystalloid infusion with regular additives or injections via the set or VAD	24 hours	Infusion fluid and sets can be more easily contaminated by frequent additions to the closed system at any point (Nichol 1999).
Parenteral nutrition	24–48 hours if system left intact. Change whole system when infusion complete.	The solution provides the ideal medium for micro-organism culture and the whole system should be replaced daily (Tait 2000).
Blood and blood products	After 12 hours or two units whichever happens first	Proteins and debris trapped in the filter lead to a high risk of bacterial colonisation (Porter 1999).
Drug infusions	Up to 24 hours	The stability and efficacy of the drug may not exceed 24 hours. The drug may react with the container such that molecules of the active component adhere to the container or set reducing the amount being infused. In addition, plasticiser used in PVC sets can leach out into the solution and be infused (Sani 1999).

will cause movement of the cannula in the vein, and phlebitis will result due to the damage to the intima. The combination of the inflammation and the repeated manipulation of the stopcock close to the insertion site significantly increase the risk of infection (see Fig. 4.3 for the suggested method for using a three-way tap on a peripheral cannula).

VADs should be well *secured* with *sterile* adhesive tape or dressings to prevent friction and movement of the device. Movement will cause phlebitis in the vein and also encourage the migration of organisms on the skin along the device and into the bloodstream (Campbell 1998). Different types of dressing are recommended depending on the device being used but any VAD should be fixed in situ with a sterile tape or dressing at the site of entry, as this constitutes a wound (Campbell & Carrington 1999). Changes must be undertaken using the aseptic technique.

Many peripheral *cannulae* used in the United Kingdom are ported devices, having access for introducing drugs or fluid through a capped opening on their dorsal surface. These ports are not covered and under the plastic snap-on cap have a cavity into which the hub of a syringe is placed to introduce drugs or fluid. There is debate about the merits and drawbacks of these types of cannulae. They enable easy administration of a small bolus of fluid without using needles to inject or breaking the system to gain access. However, they present a wide aperture through which fluid is pushed with some force, and because of their shape do not provide a flat surface for disinfection. Given their size and that the plastic caps covering them are often left loose, there is a high risk of contamination via these ports. In addition, the presence of the port often discourages the practitioner from checking the VAD site and the vein for signs of inflammation before administering drugs or fluids through it. Unless a patient requires drugs urgently (as in cardiac arrest) the port should not be used. Whenever drugs are administered via a device or its attached tubing, the vein must be inspected for inflammation and swelling and not used if either is present.

Once a VAD is inserted, fibrin adheres to it and this encourages bacteria to adhere to the cannula and avoid detection by the immune system (Weinstein 2001). It is therefore particularly important to reduce the risk and opportunity for contamination of any aspect of the IV equipment by the use of the aseptic technique and recommended practices at all times.

In-line *filters* allowing particles of not more than 0.2 microns width through, will prevent bacteria, fungi, and particles of drugs, glass and other debris being infused, prolonging the 'life' of the administration set in use. (Blood transfusion sets contain filters of 170 microns width.) However, they are expensive and, unless patients are severely immunocompromised or critically ill and dependent on numerous infusions with additives, their benefits in routine use are outweighed by their costs. Good practice should minimise the risk of particulate infusion (Johns 1996).

Signs and symptoms of infection related to VADs

Infection related to IV therapy may be either localised to the insertion site and catheter tunnel, or systemic. Systemic infections are not related to a specific area but affect the entire body. Most commonly they are experienced as bacteraemia or septicaemia. Bacteraemia refers to the presence of bacteria in the blood, often without symptoms of illness. Septicaemia also means presence of bacteria in the blood but with symptoms, and of greater severity than bacteraemia. The symptoms associated with septicaemia relate to the release of toxins into the blood by the infecting bacteria. These toxins cause the symptoms of shock and collapse described in Table 3.2. When colonised devices are used intermittently, patients may exhibit intermittent exacerbation of symptoms or rigors as 'doses' of bacteria are introduced into the bloodstream with the infusion of drugs or fluids.

For patients with central venous catheters, it is helpful to

Table 3.2 Symptoms of VAD-related infection and immediate interventions (Hart 1999)

	Signs and symptoms	Interventions
Localised infection	• pain • tenderness • inflammation at site/along device track • exudate from the site • oedema and cellulitis • fever	• remove the cannula if a peripheral catheter • swab insertion site for culture • document findings and action
Catheter-related infection	• may have no localised signs • fever may be the only sign	• if a central catheter is in situ, assume catheter-related infection unless proved otherwise • line blood cultures • peripheral blood cultures • urine, wound and sputum cultures, • insertion site swab • chest X-ray may be ordered • document findings and action • antibiotics may be commenced once cultures taken • do not remove a central venous catheter unless specifically instructed
Bacteraemia	• may be asymptomatic • intermittent fever, possibly following use of the infected device	• as above
Septicaemia	• chills • fever • malaise • tachycardia • hypotension • dehydration • rigors • cyanosis • confusion • altered consciousness • vascular shock • organ failure	• treat for shock and as symptoms arise • summon help • proceed as above

establish whether the catheter itself is the source of septi-caemia without removing the catheter. Taking blood cultures from the device and also from a peripheral vein can establish this. A catheter infection can be diagnosed if:

- catheter cultures grow a bacterium which the peripheral blood cultures do not;
- there is a higher growth in the catheter cultures than the peripheral blood;
- both sets of blood culture the same organism.

Infection and health care personnel

Handling patients' VADs and IV therapy puts health care per-sonnel at risk of infection from blood-borne organisms. Use of universal precautions, proper handwashing and aseptic tech-nique whenever indicated, should provide protection.

Needle-stick injury is a persistent problem despite recogni-tion of the hazards involved. When it does occur, the site should be made to bleed and irrigated with running water. The incident should be reported as per local policy and the occu-pational health department informed. Blood may be taken from both the patient and the injured person for hepatitis B and C and other possible infectious diseases. Continued vigi-lance in adhering to good practice and local policy should prevent needle-stick injury (Dougherty 1999). In particular, staff should be continually reminded to:

- keep up to date with health and safety procedures and the use of universal precautions;
- avoid the use of needles at all when possible (see Chapter 4 for needle-less systems);
- *never* re-sheath needles (see Chapter 4, p 109);
- *never* attempt to remove used needles from syringes;
- dispose of sharps immediately in the appropriate container;
- have sharps disposal containers where sharps are used;
- *never* attempt to retrieve an object once disposed of in a sharps container;

- ensure sharps containers are replaced before they are full;
- *never* attempt to make more room in a container;
- carefully close and dispose of used containers so they can be safely taken for incineration.

Non-sharp items including cannulae, catheters, administration sets and plastic containers may be disposed of in sacks of clinical waste for incineration.

PERIPHERAL VENOUS ACCESS DEVICES

Advantages, indications and disadvantages

Peripheral venous access is achieved usually by accessing the veins in the hands or forearms, though the feet and ankles may also be used. This provides an easy method for obtaining instant intravenous access with minimal complications. Peripheral cannulae are used for short-term drug and/or fluid administration and blood transfusion. In addition to infection, the principal problems associated with peripheral cannulae are occlusion, phlebitis, thrombophlebitis, infiltration and extravasation.

Types of cannula

Cannulae used for peripheral venous access consist of a sterile 'plastic' tube containing a sharp, hollow needle used for insertion. The device is usually made from an inert material such as Teflon or Vialon, designed to be non-irritant and reduce the level of phlebitis, platelet adhesion and bacterial colonisation as the cannula sits in the lumen of the vein. The cannula used should have the properties outlined in Table 3.3 in order to diminish the risks to the patient.

The use of ported devices is controversial, as described earlier in relation to infection. Ported cannulae enable the easy administration of drug and fluid boluses but cannot be adequately cleaned and discourage observation of the insertion site prior to administering the bolus.

Table 3.3 Advantageous features of cannulae

Advantageous features	Rationale
The narrowest, shortest device needed for the purpose	The smaller the cannula the less the trauma to the intima of the vein and the greater the flow of blood around the device diluting the infusate
Thin-walled cannula	Increases the lumen of the cannula for increased flow rate without increasing the overall width of the cannula in the lumen of the vein
Non-tapering tube	Tapering increases thrombophlebitis
Flexible material	Able to move with the patient and kink-resistant
Easily secured to the patient	Promotes patient comfort; prevents movement of the device inside the vein causing phlebitis; prevents accidental removal of the device
Secure grip	Promotes easy insertion reducing trauma to the patient and their vein
Smooth insertion	Promotes easy insertion reducing trauma to the patient and their vein
Radio-opaque components	Detectable on X-ray

As described in Table 3.3, the size of the cannula is relevant to the potential trauma it may cause the intima of the vein in which it rests. Cannula sizes relate to the cannula diameter and are stated in gauge sizes, where the increase in gauge number is inversely proportional to the diameter of the cannula. In the United Kingdom, peripheral cannula sizes are generally colour coded, as shown in Table 3.4.

Veins

The veins commonly used in peripheral cannulation are those on the dorsal surface of the hand (see Fig. 2.6), the cephalic

Table 3.4 Commonly used cannula sizes

Gauge size	Colour	Actual diameter	Flow rate	Suggested use
24 G	Yellow	0.7 mm	13 ml/hr	children
22 G	Blue	0.8 mm	31 ml/hr	drugs short-term infusions children
20 G	Pink	1 mm	54 ml/hr	drugs infusions
18 G	Green	1.2 mm	80 ml/hr	blood transfusion infusions
16 G	Grey	1.7 mm	180 ml/hr	blood transfusions large volume infusions
14 G	Brown	2 mm	270 ml/hr	blood transfusions large, rapid volume infusions

and the basilic veins up the forearm and in the antecubital fossa (see Fig. 2.7). It is preferable that cannulae are not sited over joints, so as to minimise the potential for mechanical phlebitis associated with movement of the joint and consequently movement of the cannula in the vein. However, this is not always possible and it may be necessary to immobilise the joint involved (see Bandages and Splints below).

It is important to note that veins should not be re-cannulated at a point lower than a recently used site in the same vein. Healing will be adversely affected as the vein continues to be used for infusion. Problems related to phlebitis, thrombophlebitis and infection could be exacerbated for the same reason. Consequently, using veins in the antecubital fossa for initial cannulation should be avoided, unless no others can be found and venous access is urgently required. In addition, these veins are often used for venepuncture. If they are cannulated, access for venepuncture is reduced in the short term and possibly also the long term (Dougherty 1999).

Preparation for cannulation

Prior to cannulation it is important that the patient is prepared for the procedure, psychologically as well as physically. They should be made aware of what is about to happen and the reasons for the procedure, and given the opportunity to explore their concerns or voice questions. Some patients will be very anxious about cannulation, particularly if they are repeatedly exposed to needle stabs or have had an unpleasant experience in the past. The more relaxed the patient is, the less likely the cannulation is to be traumatic.

All the equipment required should be collected in advance, and shown to the patient if indicated. The area to be cannulated should be clean or, if not, washed with soap and water before drying thoroughly. As previously described, excessive hair may be trimmed with scissors if necessary but the skin should not be shaved (p 52). The skin must then be thoroughly cleaned with an antiseptic such as 2% aqueous chlorhexidine or 70% alcohol chlorhexidine by rubbing firmly for at least a minute (Weinstein 2001). The residual solution should be allowed to dry without fanning or wiping and should not be touched again until after the cannula is in situ.

Dressings

Once the cannula is sited it needs to be secured:

- to prevent its inadvertent removal;
- to prevent mechanical phlebitis caused by movement of the cannula in and out of the vein;
- to reduce the risk of infection with movement in and out of the vein entraining organisms;
- for the patient's comfort and security.

A cannula site is a wound with direct entry to the vascular system and must be treated as any other wound with aseptic technique and sterile dressings. Choice of site dressing for peripheral cannulae should include those that:

- are sterile;
- enable visibility of the insertion site;
- prevent exogenous contamination;
- secure the cannula in situ;
- are easy to apply and remove;
- are cost effective (Campbell & Carrington 1999).

Dressings should be *changed* only if they are blood stained, have become wet or stained, or when there is fluid collecting at the insertion site. If they are dry and intact it is preferable to leave them alone. Each dressing change will open the site to exogenous infection and disturb the cannula within the vein, predisposing to phlebitis or dislodgement. If *cleaning* of the site is required then an antiseptic such as chlorhexidine should be used, as at insertion. If there is purulent exudate at the site, or signs of phlebitis, the cannula should be removed.

Sterile *gauze dressings* secured with clean tape provide a cheap dressing for cannula sites but these are not transparent and have to be removed and changed when the site is checked. Alternatively, *transparent film* dressings enable visualisation of the site and provide a secure fixing. However, some types can encourage collection of fluid around the device, which encourages bacterial proliferation, and are thus contraindicated. In addition, some not only are highly adhesive and can be difficult to apply and remove but also hold the cannula in situ with undue pressure, causing damage to the patient's skin. Campbell & Carrington (1999) found polyurethane dressings to be the most effective overall.

Bandages

It is preferable *not to bandage* cannulae. Bandages facilitate the build-up of warmth and moisture on the skin around the cannula site, encouraging infection. They also totally obscure visibility of the site and the vein. This prevents early detection of phlebitis or other complications.

However, many patients prefer to have the security offered by a light bandage to prevent snagging the device and causing movement or dislodgement of the cannula. Also, bandaging can provide a light splinting effect to discourage full movement when a vein is cannulated over a joint. If bandaging is used, it is imperative that light bandages are used and that they effectively hold the device in place without being too tight. The bandage must be removed prior to the administration of any drugs or flushes, and at least once a day so that the site may be inspected. Crepe bandages or Tubigrip can apply pressure to the area, constricting the flow of any infusion and damaging the patient's skin under the device or administration set, and should be avoided (Nichol 1999).

Splints

As with bandages, *splints should not be used* unless absolutely necessary. Long-term use of a splint can lead to nerve damage due to pressure exerted by the splint. In addition they are seldom very effective and pose a cross-infection risk. Splints are only indicated for use where a cannula is sited over a joint and the patient is unable to avoid significant movement in that joint. When used, they must be removed at least daily or whenever visualisation of the site is required if their bandaging obscures it. Splints should be disposable, or if not, thoroughly cleaned between use for different patients to prevent cross-infection (Nichol 1999).

Managing the device in situ

As previously indicated, cannulae sites should be *checked* at least daily or whenever drugs are given or infusions changed. If there is any sign of inflammation or pain the cannula should be removed.

If the cannula is not in regular use it should also be removed. However, if it is required for future use (actual or potential) it should be capped with an injectable bung and *flushed* every 12 hours to maintain patency; 2–5 ml 0.9% sodium chloride solution should be used to maintain patency in peripheral cannulae as it is effective, does not increase the risk of phlebitis, does not interact with most drugs and is cheap to use. The flush technique should be pulsatile (push-stop), removing the syringe whilst maintaining positive pressure on the plunger to prevent backflow of blood into the cannula on withdrawal (Nichol 1999).

Infusions of fluid should be administered through the appropriate *administration set*. A standard set is suitable for most infusions. Blood and blood products should be infused through a blood administration set, with the exception of platelets which require a special set supplied with the infusion. In critical care areas and in paediatrics, burette administration sets are used to enable a specific volume of fluid to be infused within a given time, avoiding accidental excess infusion. Drugs may be added to the burette and diluted before slow infusion, though thorough mixing must be ensured before the infusion is started. The rate at which sets infuse (drops per ml) is displayed on their wrappers (see Table 5.5).

When an administration set, tubing or a bung is *connected or changed* on a peripheral cannula, it is useful to place a sterile gauze square under the hub of the cannula. Pressure over the vein distal to the tip of the cannula will prevent backflow of blood when the system is opened and any blood that does leak will be caught on the gauze square. Sets should be changed as indicated in Table 3.1.

Any administration set, tubing, stopcock, syringe or injection bung connected to a cannula or administration system must be *luer-locked* in order to avoid inadvertent disconnection and the potential for haemorrhage or air embolism, and contamination of the IV system.

As the cannula is *secured* to prevent mechanical phlebitis or dislodgement, so any tubing connected to it should be for the same reasons. Tubing should be secured with tape to the patient's skin by looping the tubing so that it is unable to kink and lies flat against the patient's forearm. The tape should be adhered completely around the tubing to avoid slipping, and then adhered to the skin, away from the site dressing.

Complications

Occlusion of the device arises for the following reasons:

- backflow of blood in the cannula
  (1) because an infusion has run through or been left turned off for some time
  (2) if the device is not flushed when not being used;

- kinking of the cannula where the cannula is sited over a joint;
- kinking of the administration set or tubing if the tubing is inappropriately secured;
- the infusion is not high enough for gravity to overcome intravenous pressure;
- the cannula is a small gauge and slows the infusion;
- collection of precipitate in the device obstructs the lumen;
- venous spasm distal to the end of the cannula;
- tape or bandages are too tight, restricting flow.

Occlusion can be avoided by regular flushing before and after the administration of drugs, or daily if the cannula is not being used. Infusions should be replaced or the cannula flushed when they are complete. The cannula and tubing should be appropriately secured (see sections in this chapter on dressings, bandages and administration sets).

Venous spasm is caused by the low temperature or chemical irritation from the fluid infused, or the mechanical trauma caused by the device or infusion speed. It can be relieved by applying a warm compress, diluting the drug further, slowing the infusion or stopping it altogether.

If a cannula appears to be occluded, forceful flushing either by injection or by winding the set tubing should be avoided. This may contribute to infiltration of the infusion or push an occluding mass into the circulation and cause an embolus. The cannula should be removed otherwise there is a risk of embolus.

Infiltration occurs when fluids that are *not* vesicant or irritant (see below) are unintentionally infused into the tissues surrounding a vein instead of into the circulation. This is a very common complication of IV therapy which occurs in two ways: partial infiltration and complete infiltration. Infusion rates will slow down and resistance will be felt if a bolus of fluid is being administered with a syringe. An electronic infusion device will either alarm or continue infusing depending on its sensitivity to pressure.

(1) Partial infiltration occurs when there is constriction at, or distal to, the tip of the cannula in the vein. This restricts the flow of fluid from the cannula into the circulation. As the pressure builds up, the flow rate decreases and fluid leaks out from the vein through the device puncture site and into the surrounding tissues (see Fig. 3.2).

(2) Complete infiltration results when the cannula is displaced and the fluid infuses directly into the surrounding tissues. The cannula may either have been introduced too far through the vein lumen out of the other side of the vein, or it may have been pulled back out of the vein, but not completely removed (see Fig. 3.3 and Fig. 3.4).

Infiltration can be avoided by skilled cannulation, securing the device well and avoiding the cannulation of veins over joints whenever possible. Once infiltration is identified the cannula must be removed.

Extravasation is the infiltration of vesicant or irritant solutions into the tissues surrounding a vein, causing tissue damage and necrosis (see Fig. 3.5). Such solutions include cytotoxic drugs which are toxic to cells, electrolytes (potassium chloride when either minimally or not diluted), fluids which are of different osmolality or pH (sodium bicarbonate) from the tissues, and drugs which have a vasoconstrictive action (dopamine). This will occur in the same way as infiltration but

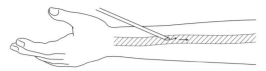

i   The cannula is infusing solution into a patent vein.

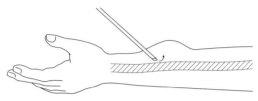

ii   The cannula tip has pulled out of the vein and is
infusing into surrounding subcutaneous tissue.

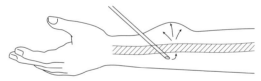

iii   The cannula tip has passed through the vein wall and is
infusing into surrounding subcutaneous tissue.

Fig. 3.2 Partial infiltration (from L. Dougherty & J. Lamb eds, *Intravenous Therapy in Nursing Practice*, Churchill Livingstone, Edinburgh, with permission)

will have a significantly more serious effect on the patient. Pain and burning will be experienced at the site, with necrosis following within 7 to 28 days. The extent of tissue damage will indicate the potential for healing, which may occur by granulation if the area is small and reasonably superficial. In this case debridement and grafting will be required, with possible loss of function. If not, amputation may be indicated (How & Brown 1998).

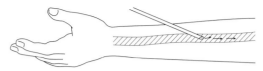

i   The cannula is infusing solution into a patent vein.

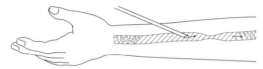

ii   Constriction has occurred around cannula. Pressure has
      increased and resistance is apparent. The valve closes and
      dilution of the infusate with blood ceases.

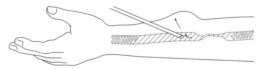

iii   Complete occlusion. Due to the pressure around the cannula,
       the cannula tip may increase the hole made on insertion, which
       will increase the likelihood of the infusate leaking into the
       surrounding tissues.

Fig. 3.3 Complete infiltration (from L. Dougherty & J. Lamb eds, *Intravenous Therapy in Nursing Practice*, Churchill Livingstone, Edinburgh, with permission)

Extravasation can be avoided by using newly sited cannulae of small gauge in large veins, avoiding sites over joints. The cannula must be checked for patency before, during and after the administration of the drug or solution. Where possible the drug should be administered in conjunction with a fast-running infusion of a compatible IV fluid for dilution. All these

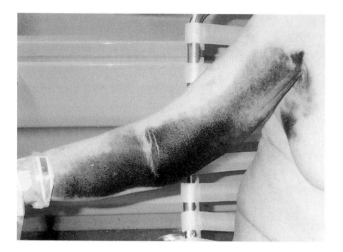

Fig. 3.4 Infiltration of a blood transfusion

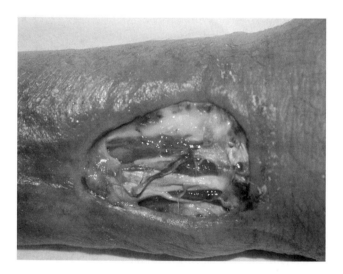

Fig. 3.5 Extensive damage following extravasation (from L. Dougherty & J. Lamb eds, *Intravenous Therapy in Nursing Practice*, Churchill Livingstone, Edinburgh, with permission)

points constitute good practice for administration of any drug intravenously, except the latter when a patient's fluid intake is restricted. Drugs causing extravasation should only be administered by those trained and experienced in doing so.

When extravasation is suspected, the infusion *must be stopped immediately*. The limb should be elevated, if possible, to reduce oedema, and the patient advised to exercise all the joints. Subsequent treatment will depend on the drug involved and the severity of the damage and should be carried out according to local guidance and policy. It is not in the scope of this text to cover the details of chemotherapy administration or extravasation. For further information see Dougherty and Lamb (1999).

Phlebitis is another common complication of IV therapy, due to inflammation of either the intima or all the layers of the vein. It is associated with pain, redness and swelling over the vein, which may develop a palpable cord (Baxter Health Care 1988 cited by Campbell 1998). It is not usually due to infection. Phlebitis is caused by irritation in the vein due to mechanical causes from the device used, or due to chemical irritation from the fluids infused or from the infusion of particles (see Fig. 3.6).

When a cannula or catheter is introduced into a vein, the traumatised tissues release chemicals in response to the injury. Among these is histamine which dilates the vein and surrounding vessels increasing blood flow to the area. It also increases permeability of the vessel wall enabling fluid and proteins to migrate to the area from the surrounding tissues. Collectively this causes the inflammation and oedema at the site. If the cannula is not removed, leucocytes migrate to the area and pus forms in the inflamed tissue, increasing the oedema locally and raising the temperature by releasing endogenous pyrogens into the bloodstream.

The risk of phlebitis can be reduced by:

- using the smallest cannula possible;
- avoiding inserting devices over joints;

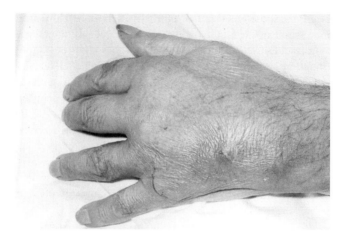

Fig. 3.6 Phlebitis

- diluting irritant drugs with compatible infusions or by having cannulae in veins with larger blood flow;
- securing devices well to avoid mechanical phlebitis;
- changing devices every 96 hours or at the earliest signs of problems (Laj 1998).

Thrombophlebitis, like phlebitis, involves inflammation of the vein, in conjunction with formation of a thrombus. It is caused by damage to vessel walls, altered blood flow (such as turbulent flow, see Chapter 2 p 35, or the flow round a device in the vein) and changes in blood chemistry (as in dehydration or sepsis). Where trauma is caused to the vessel wall, phlebitis occurs as previously described. Platelets adhere to the point of inflammation in the vessel lumen, forming a plug through which fibrin strands develop with the conversion of fibrinogen to fibrin. Blood cells are trapped in this structure forming the thrombus. Plasminogen in the circulating blood will subsequently be converted to plasmin and break down the fibrin strands so that the thrombus is eventually dissolved. In the meantime there is a danger that the thrombus will break up and emboli will be carried to the respiratory circulation or the brain, with serious consequences. However, it is more likely that septicaemia or bacterial endocarditis will result, especially if there is infection at the cannula insertion site. A thrombosed vein is permanently damaged, with hardening, loss of elasticity and abnormal blood flow (Weinstein 2001).

To avoid thrombophlebitis, similar measures should be taken as for avoiding phlebitis. Damage caused to patients' veins from repeated attempts to cannulate, use of large cannulae in small veins and the infusion of irritant solutions will all predispose to thrombophlebitis and should be avoided.

Removing a peripheral cannula

As with all other handling of IV therapy devices, removing a cannula should be an aseptic process using sterile materials for contact with the insertion site, the practitioner's hands being washed before and after the procedure. Gloves should be worn and the cannula should be gently and steadily withdrawn, then steady pressure applied to the site with sterile gauze for a minute. When bleeding has stopped, a sterile dressing or plaster should be applied and the cannula checked to ensure it is intact and has been completely removed. Ideally peripheral cannulae should be changed every 72 hours, regardless of the absence of obvious complications (Campbell 1998).

MIDLINE VENOUS CATHETERS

Midline catheters are inserted into either the basilic or cephalic vein at the antecubital fossa (see Fig. 2.7) The basilic vein is preferred as its line is straighter up the arm and it has a larger lumen. The catheters used are long (20 cm) but do not extend past the axilla. They are therefore not 'central catheters' and have advantages over peripheral cannulae without some of the disadvantages of central catheters (Dolan & Dougherty 2000).

Midline catheters can remain in situ for up to four weeks without complications and are indicated for use when:

- patients have poor peripheral venous access and cannulation is required;
- IV access is required for longer than 5 days;
- repeated cannulation would be required over some weeks causing distress to the patient and trauma to peripheral veins;
- use of a central catheter is contraindicated.

Mechanical phlebitis is a common complication of midline catheter insertion but can be treated without removal of the catheter. Warm compresses and resting the arm should resolve the phlebitis, though frequent observation is required. If the phlebitis does not resolve, the catheter would have to be removed and re-sited in the other arm.

The catheter should be secured firmly with sterile steri-strips or specially manufactured fixatives and covered with a transparent dressing to allow observation. It is preferable that the dressing is permeable to moisture; it should be changed weekly, or sooner if indicated by moisture collection or loss of adhesion.

CENTRAL VENOUS ACCESS DEVICES

Central venous access devices or 'central lines' are those whose tip lies in the superior vena cava or possibly the right atrium regardless of the site of insertion. Formerly rarely used for venous access owing to their associated risks, they are used increasingly in patients with acute clinical problems and poor peripheral venous access, or for those requiring long-term venous access for chronic conditions or long-term therapy. Their use is still associated with significant risks in both the short and the long term, and practitioners need to be fully aware of these when caring for patients with central venous access devices (CVADs) in situ.

Advantages and indications

CVADs provide access into the central venous system, that is the thoracic vessels returning blood to the right side of the heart. Blood volume and flow are highest in these vessels and the right atrium, and this enables both monitoring of the heart and blood flow dynamics as well as administration of large volumes of fluid, blood and irritant or vesicant substances into the venous system. This facilitates the dilution of the infused substances with circulating blood, significantly reducing the degree of inflammation and damage to vessels that would be caused in peripheral veins. CVADs are also used for dialysis access in acute renal failure, but this is beyond the scope of this book.

Patients who benefit from CVAD insertion include those who require:

- emergency resuscitation with fluids or blood transfusion;
- haemodynamic monitoring including central venous pressure (CVP), or right atrial pressure (RAP) and pulmonary artery pressure (PAP);
- temporary cardiac pacing with a wire passed through the CVAD into the right ventricle;
- venous access for longer than a few days or weeks and have poor peripheral veins;
- continuous cytotoxic drug infusions;
- vesicant drug infusions;
- continuous infusions of irritant drugs or fluids including parenteral nutrition (PN);
- prolonged infusions of blood or blood products;
- prolonged infusions of IV fluids or drugs;
- repeated blood sampling (Gabriel 1999).

An additional benefit of CVADs with lumens wider than 22 gauge (20G or lower) is that blood samples can be obtained from the catheter, avoiding the need for repeated venepuncture. This should only be undertaken by experienced practitioners. Guidance for this procedure can be found in Mallett & Dougherty (2000).

Disadvantages
CVADs represent a significant hazard to the patient both at the time of insertion and whilst they remain in situ. These risks are associated with infection, damage to surrounding tissues and function on insertion, phlebitis, thrombosis, occlusion, air embolism, infiltration and extravasation and damage to devices, particularly those in situ for months or years. The more common use of CVADs should not imply a reduction of risks involved in their use nor should these risks be under-estimated by the practitioner caring for the patient with a CVAD. The risks and complications associated with CVADs are described in detail in sections relating to insertion and management respectively.

Types of CVAD
Different types of device are used in different situations and for different patients' needs. Details of specific devices' characteristics may be found in Table 3.5 on pp 88–91.

Preparing the patient
Where possible, it is vital that patients are prepared psychologically as well as physically for the insertion of their CVAD; this is imperative when it is to be used in the medium to long term. The patient will be assessed and should be consulted about the need for the device, the procedures involved, and if at all possible their preferences as to the exit site and type of device used. Involving the patient by giving them information and encouraging them to make choices can promote independence in caring for the device, particularly for those who will be at home at any point during their treatment. Additionally, patients can be encouraged to ensure all practitioners who care for their device use handwashing and asepsis when dealing

with the catheter. This should reduce the risk of infection and give the patient ownership of their care (Drewett 2000).

Insertion of the device presents the following risks to the patient.

(1) *Infection* on insertion of the device is a significant risk, as already discussed. Insertion of CVADs, because of their location in the central venous system and the direct access from the protective skin into the circulation, requires strict handwashing, asepsis and the use of sterile gown, gloves and mask. Skin preparation is preferably achieved with chlorhexidine as previously described, not least because of its residual antibacterial qualities for up to 6 hours after application. The appropriate catheter for the purpose should be used and sited in the most appropriate place. Multi-lumen catheters, whilst useful, have increased risk of infection over single-lumen devices. Tunnelled or implanted catheters are associated with lower rates of infection, as are those sited in the arm or on the chest when compared with jugular or femoral sites (Pratt *et al.* 2001a,b).

(2) *Haemorrhage* is a potential risk either from trauma to vessels on attempted insertion, or if the catheter is disconnected once it is in situ. Patients' clotting times and platelet levels are checked prior to insertion of the CVAD and corrected to normal levels to prevent catastrophic haemorrhage occurring as a result of the insertion. Patients on anticoagulant therapy should have this discontinued and the line inserted when clotting times are normal. Disconnection of tubing is prevented by the use of luer locking connections.

(3) *Air embolism* on insertion is usually due to air being drawn into the central venous system through the aperture of the catheter or the needle through which it is advanced. Pressure within the thoracic cavity changes with the respiratory cycle, being equal to atmospheric pressure at the end

of expiration. As inspiration begins, the diaphragm and intercostal muscles contract, increasing the space in the thorax but creating a negative pressure within the chest. This enables air to flow into the lungs. However, if there is an alternative opening into the chest via a catheter into a central vein, air will be sucked into the chest through this as well, in this instance into the heart rather than the lungs.

This is avoidable by placing the patient flat or head down for CVAD insertion. Gravity causes the veins to engorge and this counteracts the negative pressure. Once the catheter is in situ it should be connected to a closed system using luer locks at all times, or clamped with in-line clamps before it is disconnected. Clamps should only be opened when the catheter is reconnected. All connections or bungs should be checked regularly by the practitioner caring for the patient. The use of a valved catheter will prevent air embolism once it is in situ. Some types of catheter intended for long-term use have valves at the tip which close if there is no pressure exerted by fluid flowing through them. The valve opens if there is positive pressure from drug or fluid administration, or negative pressure due to blood withdrawal.

If air embolism does occur, this constitutes a medical emergency. The patient may experience dyspnoea, chest pain, tachycardia, hypotension due to air in the cardiovascular system. Altered consciousness, visual disturbances or hemiparesis result from air embolus in the cerebral circulation. The patient should immediately be placed head down and given oxygen and medical help should be urgently summoned whilst the cause of the embolism is found and the catheter or entrance to the vein occluded. Placing the patient head down will allow the air in the heart to rise to the highest point and be trapped in the apex of the ventricles, as opposed to being circulated to the lungs and the brain.

(4) *Pneumothorax* is not an uncommon complication of CVAD insertion, particularly when the subclavian vein is cannulated (Rosen *et al.* 1992). The pleural membranes lie adjacent to the subclavian vessels; when trying to puncture the vein inadvertent puncturing of the pleura can occur. As with air embolism, if another means of air entry into the thoracic cavity is available, this time into the pleural space, air will rush into that space affecting lung expansion and gas exchange. If the pneumothorax is large the patient will become dyspnoeic and agitated, and may experience pain on breathing and require oxygen; medical help should be summoned urgently. Tension pneumothorax may lead to mediastinal shift and cardiac arrest due to pulseless electrical activity (PEA) in the heart. A chest X-ray will establish the diagnosis and a chest drain may be required to re-inflate the lung. Smaller pneumothoraces may not cause difficulty or require intervention. A pneumothorax may not be immediately obvious and may only be diagnosed on chest X-ray after the catheter has been placed in situ.

Dressings

CVAD site dressings constitute one of the most debated topics in IV therapy. The same principles apply as for peripheral cannulae. Dressings should:

- be sterile;
- enable visibility of the insertion site;
- prevent exogenous contamination;
- be permeable to water vapour;
- secure the catheter in situ;
- be easy to apply and remove;
- be cost effective.

Catheter insertion sites should be cleaned using an aseptic technique, with aqueous or alcohol-based chlorhexidine (alcohol-based antiseptics can damage the catheter over time and cause it to fracture so should not be allowed to soak the catheter) and preferably dressed in transparent, moisture-permeable adhesive film dressings, though gauze and tape may also be used (Pratt *et al.* 2001a). These should be changed 24 hours after catheter insertion and then weekly, or more often if no longer providing an effective seal, if not securing the device or if there is moisture collecting under it. The site should be cleaned with chlorhexidine when the dressing is changed and swabbed if there is purulent exudate or inflammation at the insertion site.

Non-tunnelled and peripherally inserted central catheters (PICCs) will always require dressings. PICCs should be secured with special securing devices or sterile steristrips then covered with a transparent, semi-permeable adhesive dressing film. If used intermittently, the hub of a PICC can be sealed under a transparent adhesive dressing as can the entry site (with a continuous film) to seal the site and catheter hub, thus enabling the patient to shower or bathe.

Cuffed tunnelled catheters should not require dressing once the cuff has been infiltrated by growing tissue (approximately one week after insertion). The secured cuff provides a barrier to organisms trying to track down the tunnel the catheter is lying in.

Implanted ports (see Table 3.5) should only require dressing until the insertion site wound is healed. However, if a patient with an implanted port requires a continuous infusion, sterile gauze can be placed under the needle to avoid pressure damage to the underlying skin. The needle, administration set and gauze can then be covered with a dressing.

Complications
Ongoing complications once the catheter is in situ may be equally hazardous to the patient but are often avoidable with good practice.

(1) *Infection* is always a major hazard for patients with CVADs and the use of strict handwashing and asepsis in handling

the catheter is imperative at all times as the catheter provides a direct route into the central circulatory system. Ryder (2001) described the development of a bacterial 'biofilm' that builds up on surfaces such as CVADs and is related to the development of catheter-related infections. Asepsis and regular handwashing are preventative measures which offer the principal defence against complications of catheter-related sepsis.

The more a central catheter is manipulated the more likely it is to become infected and cause septicaemia in the patient. Connections, bungs, ports and the catheter hub should all be cleaned with chlorhexidine or povidone-iodine before they are used (Pratt *et al*. 2001a). As with peripheral cannulae, the use of three-way stopcocks or extension sets should be avoided or kept to a minimum as they provide increased potential for contamination by virtue of their difficulty to clean and the manipulation they require. If a patient with a CVAD in situ develops a pyrexia, the cause should be assumed to be related to the catheter until proven otherwise (see Table 3.2).

Some CVADs are now coated with antimicrobial agents to discourage colonisation of the catheter and these may be used effectively for patients at high risk of infection (Pratt *et al*. 2001b).

(2) *Chemical phlebitis* is rarely associated with CVADs because their tips are situated in an area with a high volume of blood flow.

Mechanical phlebitis can occur within seven days when devices are sited in small veins and blood flow around the device is restricted (as with PICCs). This should resolve with warm compresses, but if still problematic after a week, infection may be suspected (see above).

(3) *Thrombophlebitis* in central veins relates to the initial trauma to the vein on insertion of the catheter and to the presence of catheter. The larger and more rigid the catheter the higher the risk of thrombophlebitis. Throm-

bosis will form (as described on p 44) at the site but fragments may migrate to distant capillary beds in the lungs. The patient may experience redness and inflammation at the site of entry into the vein, pain and oedema and pyrexia. If severe, there may be pain and swelling down the arm on the side the device was inserted, or neck distension and facial swelling. The arm on the affected side may appear pale or mottled.

Heparin, urokinase or other thrombolytic agents may be infused through the catheter to treat thrombosis in long-term catheters (Weinstein 2001).

(4) *Occlusion* of a CVAD may be *intraluminal*, commonly due to obstruction of its lumen with a blood clot, or the precipitation or crystallisation of infused substances. Both infusion and withdrawal will be increasingly difficult and may become impossible. Obstruction of the catheter from outside its lumen – *extraluminal* – can also occur and is characterised by the catheter being open to infusion but not to withdrawal of blood. This is due to:

- poor positioning or migration of the catheter tip into a smaller vein;
- migration of the catheter out of the circulatory system to the surrounding tissues;
- anatomical obstruction by the clavicle, enlarged lymph nodes or radiation damage to tissues in the area;
- formation of a fibrin sheath around the catheter which occludes the tip on negative pressure.

Prevention is achieved by appropriate infusion of drugs and fluids to avoid precipitation, and flushing of all the catheter lumens before and after use with 0.9% sodium chloride to maintain patency. It is recommended that CVAD lumens are flushed with a push-stop, push-stop method and that they are clamped whilst a positive pressure is being exerted through the syringe. Some injection ports are designed to achieve this. There is no consensus about the frequency or type of flush to use (0.9% sodium chloride or heparinised saline) and this is often dictated by local policy. Some catheters are specifically manufactured to avoid the need to flush the lumens between uses. Practitioners should familiarise themselves with manufacturers' recommendations for the particular product the patient has in situ, and act accordingly.

If occlusion is suspected, an experienced practitioner should be consulted before any attempt is made to unblock the lumen. Initially, aspiration may be attempted to ascertain the type of occlusion and to free small clots in the catheter. Syringes of 10 ml volume or more should be used, as smaller ones will create too high a pressure and may rupture the catheter. Depending on the cause of the obstruction, agents may be instilled down the lumen to restore patency. Removal of the device is usually a last resort.

(5) *Air embolus* is avoided in valved catheters, and in open-tipped catheters should be avoided by clamping the lumen prior to opening the system and ensuring all attachments or bungs are securely luer-locked. When an infusion is being given into an open-tipped CVAD from a rigid (glass) container with an air inlet to facilitate flow, the practitioner caring for the patient must be vigilant in stopping the infusion before there is a chance for air to run into the catheter from the empty infusion set. All equipment connected to CVADs must be luer-locked together to avoid disconnection and subsequent air embolus, or haemorrhage. Closed luer-locked bungs are often fitted to the end of CVAD lumens. A latex diaphragm in the bung seals when an infusion set or syringe is not attached to the catheter.

(6) *Infiltration and extravasation* (see p 67) of fluid to the surrounding tissues occur relatively infrequently with CVADs. Patients and practitioners should be alert for signs

of pain, redness and swelling at the insertion site of the catheter or along the track of a tunnelled device either during or after an infusion. Extravasation may occur due to damage to the catheter, migration of the catheter tip, backtracking of the infusion from the vein out of the insertion site and into the surrounding tissues, or dislodgement of the needle from the port of an implanted CVAD (portacath). Flushing the catheter with 0.9% sodium chloride before commencing an infusion or administering drugs should indicate potential difficulty. If extravasation or infiltration are thought to have occurred, the infusion must be stopped immediately and help summoned (see p 67).

(7) *Damaged catheters* can result from the use of 'toothed' clamps (Spencer Wells forceps) on the catheter, repeated clamping on a long-term catheter, wear and tear of the catheter in the portion exiting the patient, repeated use of alcohol-based antiseptic solutions, or accidental use of scissors on the catheter. When a non-valved catheter is damaged on the external end, it should immediately be clamped distal to the damaged part. External portions of CVADs for medium- or long-term use can be repaired according to manufacturers' instructions, though precautions should be taken to avoid damaging them, including avoiding unnecessary manipulation, using non-toothed clamps on lines without valves, and avoiding using scissors near the catheter.

Internally, catheters can be ruptured by the use of excessive pressure in flushing, or as a result of 'pinch-off syndrome' where the catheter is pinched between the clavicle and the first rib. Rarely, the tip of a catheter can be severed whilst in situ and migrate into the right side of the heart or the pulmonary artery. When flushing the lumens or giving drugs, syringes of 10 ml volume or more should be used to avoid a high pressure build-up in the lumen, which could lead to its rupture. Damaged PICCs may be replaced at the same site with the use of a guidewire through the old catheter and then threading the new catheter over the guidewire when the damaged one has been removed. Confirmation of the problem and attempts at repair should be made only by experts in CVAD placement and management.

Measuring central venous pressure

With a central venous catheter in situ, central venous pressure (CVP) can be monitored by measuring the pressure exerted by the blood in the right atrium or superior vena cava. This is achieved using a water manometer connected to the central catheter or with an electronic transducer in critical care areas. CVP measurement is indicated in patients who are critically ill to monitor:

- fluid balance;
- the circulating volume;
- the degree of heart failure.

Comparative measurements and trends are generally more useful than individual measurements. For accuracy, measurements must always be taken from the same point unless electronically transduced. The sternal angle or mid-axilla may be used as the measuring point, but not both, as there is a difference of 5 cm H_2O between them. The point used should be marked on the patient, documented and communicated to different practitioners when care is handed over so that there is consistency between readings and the trend is representative of the patient's haemodynamic status.

For manual readings the patient should be laid flat and the manometer's zero level aligned horizontally with the sternal notch or mid-axilla. If the patient cannot lie flat the mid-axilla site is used. The manometer is filled with crystalloid solution almost to the top of the tubing (see Fig. 3.7) and then the level in the tubing is allowed to fall until equal to the level in the superior vena cava (at the tip of the central catheter). When the fluid level stabilises (it will move up and down around a

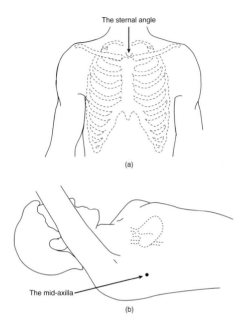

Fig. 3.7 Measuring CVP (from J. Mallett & L. Dougherty, *Royal Marsden Manual of Clinical Nursing Procedures* 5th edn, Blackwell Science, Oxford, with permission)

mid-point with respiration) the measurement is recorded, the infusion resumed and the patient made comfortable.

Removing a CVAD

Prior to removing a CVAD, the type of device in situ must be confirmed and the appropriate specific actions taken to safely remove it by the most experienced and appropriate health care professional.

The general principles of removing a central catheter are common to all types and that is to avoid air embolism and subsequent contamination of the site (using aseptic technique):

- prepare the patient for the procedure;
- if possible the patient should lie flat or head down as for insertion, to engorge the central veins and reduce the risk of air embolism using gravity;
- clean the area with aqueous chlorhexidine if exudate is present;
- remove sutures or fixings (such as steristrips);
- ask the patient to breathe in and hold their breath (particularly important if they are unable to lie down);
- pull the catheter gently and firmly until it is removed;
- apply pressure to the site using sterile gauze for several minutes and allow the patient to breathe;
- apply a sterile, occlusive dressing to the site for 72 hours;
- check that the removed catheter is intact and inform medical staff if not;
- send the tip for culture and sensitivity if infection is suspected, if the patient is pyrexial or if the patient is immunocompromised or immunosuppressed.

Specific requirements for individual types of device can be found in Table 3.5.

Table 3.5 Characteristics of commonly used CVADs (Dougherty & Lamb 1999, Weinstein 2001)

Name of central catheter	Vein insertion site	Skin exit site	Types	Lumens	Dwell time	Advantages	Disadvantages	Removal
Percutaneous	Internal jugular	Left or right neck	Open-ended (free back-flow up catheter)	Single, double or triple	Days	• Easy, immediate access for surgery or emergencies.	• Uncomfortable • Difficult to secure due to position • Mechanical phlebitis due to position • High risk of contamination • Risk of air embolism in open-ended catheters	As soon as no longer required or replaced. Not for long-term use.
	External jugular	Left or right neck	Open-ended	As above	Days	• Low risk of pneumothorax	• As above • Difficult to cannulate due to anatomy	As indicated
	Subclavian vein	Upper left or right chest under clavicle	Open-ended	Single, double or triple. Lumens have different exit sites to	Up to 3 weeks	• Convenient position for CVAD • Easy to secure and dress	• Insertion hazardous due to proximity to heart, lungs and major vessels and nerves	As indicated

	Site	Catheter	Lumens	Duration	Advantages	Comments
					avoid mixing of drugs and fluids at the point of exit (see Fig. 3.11).	• Chest X-ray to confirm tip position and exclude pneumothorax • Risk of air embolism in open-ended catheters • As indicated • Apply heat to the vein to reduce spasm, if removal is difficult • Try again later
PICC (see Fig. 3.10)	Basilic preferably, cephalic or median cubital (bifurcates to the brachial and cephalic) (see Fig. 2.6)	Open-ended or valved	Single or double	Up to several months	• Do not need to lie flat for insertion • Fewer major complications • Easily replaced • Well tolerated	• Chest X-ray to confirm tip position and exclude pneumothorax • Can 'kink' if placed low in antecubital fossa • Mechanical phlebitis not uncommon • Risk of air embolism in open-ended catheters
	Antecubital fossa preferably in the non-dominant arm					
Tunnelled (see Figs 3.8 & 3.9)	Subclavian vein	Often 'cuffed' with Dacron in subcutaneous	Single, double or triple	Months or years	• Tunnelling reduces infection • Cuffed catheters	• Need sedation and local anaesthetic or general
	Right or left chest wall several cm below clavicle					• Removed by specially trained practitioners • Surgical

89

Table 3.5 *Continued*

Name of central catheter	Vein insertion site	Skin exit site	Types	Lumens	Dwell time	Advantages	Disadvantages	Removal
			portion to prevent dislogement. Valved or open-ended.			secured without sutures • No need for dressing once sites healed	anaesthetic to insert • Chest X-ray to confirm tip position and exclude pneumothorax • Risk of air embolism in open-ended catheters	excision at point of cuff for most cuffed catheters using local anaesthetic • Wound sutured and sterile dressing applied • Pressure to skin exit site with sterile gauze. Apply sterile dressing
Implanted ports (see Fig. 3.12)	Subclavian vein, jugular veins, cephalic vein or femoral vein	None. Accessed via needle through skin over the injection port.	Valved or open-ended	Single or double. Each lumen has separate injection port with a reservoir covered by	Months or years	• Totally internal system almost eliminates infection risk • No	• Usually inserted under general anaesthetic • Chest X-ray to confirm tip position	• Cut-down method using local or general anaesthetic

a silastic membrane.

catheter care required
- Less risk of altered body image
- Only needs flushing monthly if not in regular use

and exclude pneumothorax
- Discomfort accessing the port through the skin
- Risk of extravasation if needle does not access reservoir under membrane
- Regular assessment required
- Use 10 ml syringes or larger to avoid rupture of device
- Membrane can leak after multiple punctures (up to 2000)

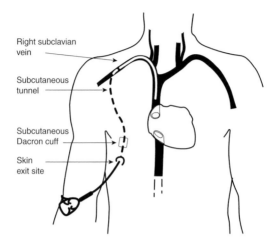

Right subclavian vein

Subcutaneous tunnel

Subcutaneous Dacron cuff

Skin exit site

Fig. 3.8 Anatomical position of a tunnelled CVAD

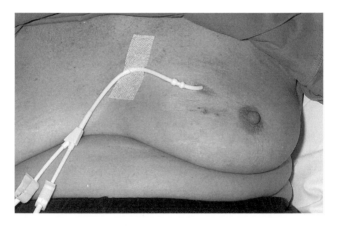

Fig. 3.9 Tunnelled CVAD in situ (Hickman line)

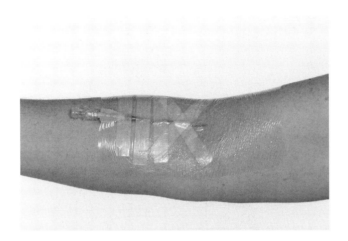

Fig. 3.10 PICC

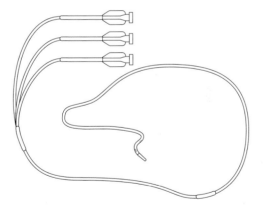

Fig. 3.11 Triple lumen CVAD showing exit sites of each lumen

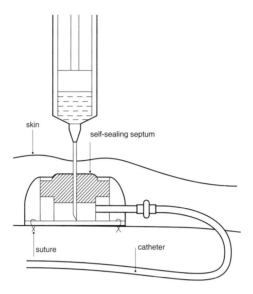

Fig. 3.12 Portacath system showing percutaneous access to the injection port (from The Medical Illustration Department, Royal Marsden Hospital NHS Trust, with permission)

Key points

- Vascular access devices, particularly central venous catheters, hold significant risks for patients, including infection, phlebitis, thrombophlebitis and embolism (air or particulate)

- Adhering to principles of handwashing and asepsis at all times is crucial in the prevention of potentially fatal VAD-associated infection

- Patient care must include strategies to minimise damage to patients' veins

- The appropriate device must be used for the required purpose and not left in situ for any longer than required

- Peripheral cannulae should ideally be changed after 72 hours and must be removed at the earliest sign of inflammation, occlusion or infiltration/extravasation

- Equipment used for infusion and drug administration should minimise handling of the device and 'breaking' the closed system, but must also be changed regularly to prevent contamination or chemical alteration of drug infusions

- Devices must be kept patent using a push-stop flushing technique when not in constant use

- VADs must be secured and the insertion point and vein checked daily and whenever drugs are administered or infusions changed

- The risks of inserting CVADs must be understood and complications checked for, including infection, haemorrhage, pneumothorax and embolism

- Nothing should be administered through a CVAD until its tip position is confirmed as appropriate

- Practitioners should be familiar with the characteristics of their patients' VADs and know how to care for them accordingly

- CVADs should only be removed by a competent practitioner when a decision has been agreed by the team responsible for the patient's care

REFERENCES

Baxter Health Care (1988) *Principles and Practice of Intravenous Therapy.* Baxter Health Care Limited, Compton, Berks. Cited in L. Campbell (1998) IV-related phlebitis; complications and length of hospital stay 2. *British Journal of Nursing* **7**(22), 1364–1373.

Campbell, H. & Carrington, M. (1999) Peripheral intravenous cannula dressings; advantages and disadvantages. *British Journal of Nursing* **8**(21), 1420–1427.

Campbell, L. (1998) IV-related phlebitis; complications and length of hospital stay 2. *British Journal of Nursing* **7**(22), 1364–1373.

Dolan, S. & Dougherty, L. (2000) Vascular access devices: insertion and management. In: J. Mallett & L. Dougherty, *Royal Marsden*

Manual of Clinical Nursing Procedures 5th edn. Blackwell Science, Oxford.

Dougherty, L. (1999) Obtaining peripheral venous access. In: L. Dougherty & J. Lamb eds, *Intravenous Therapy in Nursing Practice*. Churchill Livingstone, Edinburgh.

Dougherty, L. & Lamb J. eds (1999) *Intravenous Therapy in Nursing Practice*. Churchill Livingstone, Edinburgh.

Drewett, S.R. (2000) Complications of central venous catheters: nursing care. *British Journal of Nursing* **9**(8), 466–477.

Gabriel, J. (1999) Long-term central venous access. In: L. Dougherty & J. Lamb eds, *Intravenous Therapy in Nursing Practice*. Churchill Livingstone, Edinburgh.

Hart, S. (1999) Infection control. In: L. Dougherty & J. Lamb eds, *Intravenous Therapy in Nursing Practice*. Churchill Livingstone, Edinburgh.

How, C. & Brown, J. (1998) Extravasation of cytotoxic chemotherapy from peripheral veins. *European Journal of Oncology Nursing* **2**(1), 51–58.

Johns, T. (1996) Intravenous filters: panacea or placebo? *Journal of Clinical Nursing* **5**(1), 3–6.

Laj, K.K. (1998) Safety of prolonging peripheral cannula and IV tubing use from 72 hours to 96 hours. *American Journal of Infection Control* **26**(1), 66–70.

Maki, D.G. & Ringer, M. (1991) Risk factors for infusion-related phlebitis with small peripheral venous catheters. *Annals of Internal Medicine* **114**(10), 845–854.

Maki, D.G., Ringer, M. & Alvarado, C.J. (1991) Prospective, randomised trial of povidone iodine, alcohol and Chlorhexidine for prevention of infection associated with central venous catheters and arterial catheters. *The Lancet* **338**, 339–343.

Mallett, J. & Dougherty, L. (2000) *Royal Marsden Manual of Clinical Nursing Procedures* 5th edn. Blackwell Science, Oxford.

Nichol, M. (1999) Safe administration and management of peripheral intravenous therapy. In: L. Dougherty & J. Lamb eds, *Intravenous Therapy in Nursing Practice*. Churchill Livingstone, Edinburgh.

Nystrom, B., Larsen, S.O., Dankert, J., Daschner, F., Greco, D., Gronroos, P., Jepsen, O.B., Lystad, A., Meers, P.D. & Rotter, M. (1983) Bacteraemia in surgical patients with intravenous devices. *Journal of Hospital Infection Control* **4**(4), 338–349.

Philpott-Howard, J. & Casewell, M. (1994) *Hospital Infection Control: Policies and Practical Procedures*. W.B. Saunders, London.

Porter, H. (1999) Blood transfusion therapy. In: L. Dougherty & J. Lamb eds, *Intravenous Therapy in Nursing Practice*. Churchill Livingstone, Edinburgh.

Pratt, R., Pellowe, C., Harper, P., Loveday, H. & Robinson, N. (2001a) Preventing infections associated with central venous catheters. *Nursing Times* **97**(15), 36–39.

Pratt, R., Pellowe, C.M., Loveday, H.P., Robinson, N. & Smith, G.W. (2001b) *Phase 1: The Development of National Evidence-based Guidelines for preventing Hospital Acquired Infections in England associated with the use of Central Venous Catheters: technical report.* http://www.epic.tvu.ac.uk/epicphase/epic1.html

Rosen, M., Latto, P. & Ng, S. (1992) *Handbook of Percutaneous Central Venous Catheterisation*. W.B. Saunders, Philadelphia.

Ryder, M. (2001) The role of biofilm in vascular catheter-related infections. *New Developments in Vascular Disease* **2**(2), 15–25.

Sani, M.H. (1999) Pharmacological aspects of intravenous drug therapy. In: L. Dougherty & J. Lamb eds, *Intravenous Therapy in Nursing Practice*. Churchill Livingstone, Edinburgh.

Tait, J. (2000) Nursing management. In: H. Hamilton ed., *Total Parenteral Nutrition: a Practical Guide for Nurses*. Churchill Livingstone, Edinburgh.

Weinstein, S.M. (2001) *Plumer's Principles and Practice of Intravenous Therapy* 7th edn. Lippincott, Philadelphia.

ADDITIONAL TEXT

Dakin, M.J. & Yentis, S.M. (1998) Latex allergy: a strategy for management. *Anaesthesia* **53**, 774–781.

WEBSITES

National evidence-based guidelines for preventing hospital-acquired infections including care of CVCs
http://www.epic.tvu.ac.uk/epicphase/epic1.html

Information about IV therapy and care
http://www.ivteam.com

Managing IV Therapy Safely

4

INTRODUCTION

Intravenous access provides a direct route for treating patients with drugs and fluids, as well as for monitoring their haemodynamic status. Advances in medical equipment technology and drug treatments have led to a significant increase in the use of the intravenous route for medication in recent decades. With this increase there have been developments in practitioners' understanding and skills in the care of patients having IV therapy. However, the frequency with which the IV route is now used in all areas of health care means that almost all nurses, and many practitioners of other disciplines, need to have fundamental knowledge and competence to administer intravenous drugs safely to patients in their area of practice. This chapter details the practical, 'how to' approaches to IV drug administration and will give some insight into the benefits and dangers of using this route for drug administration. The chapter covers:

❏ the pros and cons of venous access for drug administration;
❏ preparing to administer IV therapy;
❏ anaphylaxis;
❏ reconstitution and preparing drugs for IV administration;
❏ administration of IV drugs;
❏ pumps;
❏ documentation.

PROS AND CONS OF VENOUS ACCESS FOR DRUG ADMINISTRATION

The *advantages* to patients of using the intravenous route include:

- a means of rapid drug administration with immediate effect;
- a painless way of administering drugs by injection;
- a route for administering drugs that would otherwise damage surrounding tissues;
- a route for administering drugs that would be altered in, or could not be absorbed from, the gut;
- a means of achieving constant plasma levels of a drug, avoiding the variables affecting uptake from the gut or tissues;
- a route for correcting fluid and electrolyte imbalances or administering nutrition when the gut is not functional.

The *disadvantages* of using the intravenous route also give an indication of the implications for care:

- once administered intravenously, a drug *cannot be retrieved* and its effect will be experienced rapidly;
- 'speed shock' can result when drugs are given too quickly; toxic levels in the plasma cause collapse and possible cardiac arrest;
- drugs may react with other compounds in solution and precipitation of particles can occur, leading to embolism if infused;
- drugs can be altered in solution or in certain containers, to become less active or toxic, with the result that they may not be therapeutic or may even be harmful if infused;
- venous access provides a direct route of entry into the body for micro-organisms, thus posing a significant risk of infection;
- cannulating a vein and administering substances into it is likely to cause irritation to the vein, risking phlebitis and thrombophlebitis;
- administration is time-consuming.

Giving drugs intravenously is potentially dangerous, principally because of the drugs' rapid transport and action, but also because of the less immediate complications including infection, thrombophlebitis or embolism. However, the route is therapeutically highly effective and with sound knowledge and skills practitioners will be able to enhance patients' therapy with minimal risk or complication.

PREPARING TO ADMINISTER IV THERAPY

Whatever the drug or infusion to be given, there are common steps to consider and complete in preparing to administer IV therapy to patients.

Before administering IV therapy

Practitioners administering drugs intravenously must have undertaken suitable education and training in the theoretical aspects of IV therapy and have been deemed competent after a period of supervised practice. Sound knowledge of the drugs likely to be administered to patients in their area of practice is important so that prescriptions may be administered professionally, questioning possible anomalies before an inaccurate prescription is administered and causes harm to the patient. Local policy for IV therapy must be followed and some institutions have lists of drugs that may be given by the intravenous route. Non-medical practitioners giving drugs not on such a list would not be covered by their employers' vicarious liability in the event of an adverse incident (see Chapter 1).

Anaphylaxis

The administration of some drugs can cause allergic reactions in some patients, and these can vary from being mild to life-threatening. It is important practitioners understand the pathophysiology of anaphylaxis before developing their practice in intravenous drug therapy. The speed at which IV therapy is administered induces responses both therapeutic and detrimental, responses which may occur very rapidly, and practitioners must be able to respond appropriately and quickly to patients' adverse reactions.

When an 'allergic' response occurs, the patient's immune system responds to an antigen (the substance introduced which causes the allergic reaction; a drug such as ampicillin for example) in one of two ways.

(1) *Type 1: Immediate hypersensitivity or true anaphylaxis*

On first administration of the drug, there is no visible reaction. However, particles of the antigen (the drug) have been identified by the B and T cells, and antibodies to the drug have been produced. These antibodies wait, bound to mast cells, for the next exposure to the antigen. When this happens (for example with the second dose of a five-day course of IV ampicillin) the antigen binds to the antibodies and this provokes a chain reaction where histamine is released. Within 5 to 30 minutes, the patient may experience:
  - pruritis (itching);
  - erythema (red rash);
  - wheezing and dyspnoea as the bronchioles constrict;
  - vomiting, abdominal cramps and diarrhoea;
  - vasodilation with falling blood pressure and increased heart rate;
  - laryngeal oedema and airway obstruction;
  - cardiac arrhythmias;
  - death, if intervention for the above is not immediate.

(2) *Type II: Antibody-dependent cytotoxicity*

This reaction can occur on the patient's first exposure to the allergen or drug. The drug combines with free antibodies in the circulation and attaches to tissues. The antibody–antigen combined molecule attracts complement, a series of chemicals which destroy the surrounding cells. The effects on the patient are the same as those described for Type I reactions (Nowack & Handford 1999).

The release of chemicals by the immune system has immediate and widespread effects when the 'antigen' is a drug administered IV. The potential consequence of anaphylaxis is respiratory arrest and vascular shock, the development of which is represented in Fig. 4.1.

Management of an anaphylactic or allergic reaction should be directed to the symptoms experienced by the patient. Practitioners should:

- summon help;
- stop the infusion if it is still in progress;
- maintain the patient's airway, administering oxygen;
- monitor breathing (rate, colour and oxygen saturation);

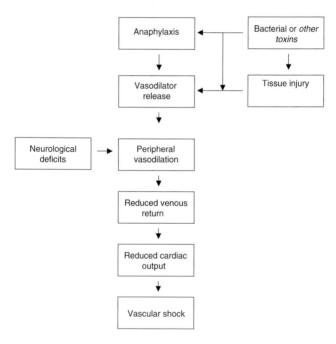

Fig. 4.1 Pathogenesis of vascular shock precipitated by anaphylaxis (from T.J. Nowack & A.G. Handford, *Essentials of Pathophysiology* 2nd edn, WCB McGraw-Hill, Boston, with permission)

- monitor circulation (heart rate and blood pressure);
- maintain intravenous access for the administration of adrenaline (epinephrine) and antihistamines, possibly also hydrocortisone when help arrives, according to local policy.

Severe anaphylaxis can be avoided by ensuring that:

- patients' allergies are recorded and that information is clearly documented, communicated and acted on;
- patients are observed during drug administration;
- practitioners involved in IV therapy are instructed and competent in anaphylaxis recognition and management.

Do the 'right' thing

Careful checking of all the elements involved in drug administration is crucial to reducing error and potential harm to patients. Single-person checking and administration is permitted in a number of areas other than controlled drug administration. However, whether one or two people are involved in checking drugs, *both* should check independently and reach agreement about the elements of the process, rather than one relying on the other to do so. Regardless of perceptions about experience, hierarchy or expertise, any practitioner involved in drug administration should be satisfied in their own mind that *all* the elements are correct before agreeing with another.

Preparation of drugs for IV administration should ideally take place in a quiet environment with minimal disturbances or distractions. This is necessary for two reasons:

- to reduce the likelihood of error due to interruptions;
- a 'clean' area with necessary equipment and handwashing facilities will aid the safe preparation of drugs, minimising contamination of the drug or personnel in the vicinity of their preparation.

The 'right' thing involves checking that five elements of a drug administration procedure are correct (Clayton 1987).

The right patient

The prescription being administered should be checked for the patient's identity and this should correspond with the patient to whom the drug will be given. Patients without identity bands should be asked their name and date of birth. Those in hospital should be given an identity band as a matter of urgency. Any allergies the patient may have relating to the drug being given should be established and recorded.

The right drug

The prescription needs to be checked for accuracy. The prescription must be clearly written, dated appropriately (covering the date on which it is being given) and signed by the prescriber. Generic drug names should be used, for example ranitidine as opposed to Zantac, and the dose, route, frequency and times for administration stated.

The drug in question must be checked to establish:

- it is the drug prescribed;
- it is suitable for IV use;
- it is an appropriate quantity;
- it is within the expiry date;
- its compatibility with any existing infusion so that it may be administered safely;
- if it needs reconstituting, or further dilution;
- the diluent to be used is compatible and checked similarly to the drug itself.

It is a good idea not to remove different solutions from their packaging until use. Having unmarked containers full of ampoules of different fluids or drugs can lead to error. Labelled boxes may be emptied into the wrong containers, or positions of unmarked containers changed, resulting in the wrong ampoule being used by someone who makes an assumption about what it should be, because that is what is usually in that place.

The right dose
There are two aspects to checking the dose. Firstly, the practitioner must recognise an appropriate dose of the drug to be administered and query the prescription if it appears to be out of the usual range. Secondly, on preparation of the drug, the prescribed dose must be drawn up for administration. At times this will involve calculations. It is imperative that practitioners are competent at mathematical calculations in order that the 'right dose' is administered (for further information on calculations see Chapter 6). As described earlier, where two people are involved in checking the drug and the calculation of the dose, they should both do the calculation and compare answers, rather than one person 'agreeing' the other's maths is correct. It is important to be able to show how the answer was achieved, particularly when working with students or inexperienced practitioners, though they too should do the maths and compare their answer.

The right time
The drug must be given at the prescribed time to maintain the appropriate therapeutic serum levels. It is important to check whether or not the patient has already had the intended dose of the drug, if at all possible. If the prescription has not been signed as given, double doses may be given inadvertently.

The right route
As previously mentioned, it must be established that the drug is suitable for IV use and the dose appropriate for IV use. If this does not appear to be the case the prescription should be checked with the prescriber and a pharmacist. Once the appropriate drug is ready for administration, the practitioner giving it must check that they *are giving the drug intravenously* and into the most appropriate device (if there is more than one). This is crucial because if, for example, a patient has both epidural and intravenous infusions, it is essential to check that the

intravenous infusion syringe is attached to the venous access. Changing the entire infusion apparatus every time the infusion syringe is changed facilitates this. Of course, this should be avoided, because the site of the device should be checked for signs of oedema, inflammation and patency every time the infusion is changed.

RECONSTITUTING AND PREPARING IV DRUGS FOR IV ADMINISTRATION

Some drugs are packaged ready for administration, others require dilution and some require reconstitution from powder to liquid form. It is important to undertake this aspect of IV therapy as carefully as the direct administration of the drug, to avoid complications. Cytotoxic drugs require special precautions for their preparation, which is beyond the scope of this book (see Additional Texts and Websites lists p 155).

Work should be undertaken on a clean surface that is easily disinfected, with equipment and handwashing facilities nearby:

- clean the work surface with 70% alcohol spray and allow it to dry;
- all the equipment and the drug required should be collected, including a clean tray in which to carry the prepared drug and equipment to the patient;
- check the drug, and, if these are required, diluent and flush solutions, and check the prescription as described above;
- check all the equipment and its packaging are intact, sterile and within the date for shelf life.

Hands must be washed and dried thoroughly and an alcohol hand rub used for decontamination.

Preparing vials of powder

Principal hazards encountered with reconstituting vials of powder are:

(1) Particle contamination due to the incomplete dissolving of the powder in the diluent or coring of the rubber stopper in the vial by the needles piercing it (Weinstein 2001).

(2) Spraying of the drug into the atmosphere by formation of an aerosol when the drug is being reconstituted and drawn up under pressure.

(3) Splashing of the drug onto the practitioner's skin or the surrounding area.

Some drugs are dispensed with manufacturers' instructions and equipment for reconstitution, which should be followed. Otherwise hazards may be avoided or minimised by careful use of the recommended techniques.

(1) Snap the lid off the container and rub the container's rubber stopper firmly with an alcohol wipe; allow it to dry without blowing or blotting it to prevent contamination.

(2) Vent the bottle with a 21 gauge needle (green) if a needle-less system is not being used. Always keep the vent needle tip *above the fluid level* in the vial to avoid fluid leaking from the vial (see Fig. 4.2).

(3) Draw up the appropriate diluent for the drug with syringe and 23 gauge needle (blue) and add it to the vial gently, running it down the side of the vial. Make sure that the powder is wet before shaking the vial. If not, powder could be released into the atmosphere.

(4) Having removed the diluent needle and syringe, cover the vent needle with an alcohol swab and gently shake the vial to dissolve the powder.

(5) Ensure that the powder is dissolved and check the solution is clear and free from particles. *Do not use it* if this is not the case, and contact the pharmacist.

(6) Clean the top of the rubber stopper with alcohol, as before, and withdraw the required volume of fluid. Check the syringe for particles, including any rubber that may have been 'cored' out of the rubber stopper by the needles (discard the solution and start again if these are present).

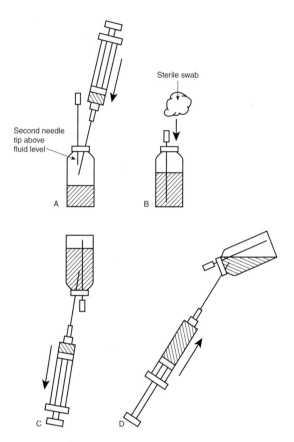

Fig. 4.2 Technique for reconstituting a vial of powder to avoid environmental exposure (from J. Mallett & L. Dougherty, *Royal Marsden Manual of Clinical Nursing Procedures* 5th edn, Blackwell Science, Oxford, with permission)

(7) The risk of coring can be reduced by inserting needles into rubber stoppers with the bevel up, and at a 45° angle, moving the needle to the 90° angle when it is almost completely inserted (Dougherty 2000a).

(8) Tap the syringe with the vial inverted and re-inject air into the vial to remove it from the syringe.

Do not spray air into the atmosphere, or re-sheath the needle and then expel the air. Firstly, this forms an aerosol and introduces the drug into the atmosphere. Secondly, re-sheathing needles with two hands (syringe and needle in one, sheath in the other) should be avoided. If a practitioner is used to re-sheathing needles, even though they think they only do so with clean ones, they are at increased risk of needlestick injury with clean **or** contaminated needles. A re-sheathing device can be used before removing the needle. Alternatively a one-handed technique can be used to cover the needle before removing it, where the practitioner holds the syringe and needle in one hand and inserts the needle into its sheath.

(9) Replace the needle with a 25 gauge needle (orange) or other needle-less device for administration of the drug.

(10) Discard used needles into a sharps container.

Preparing ampoules of powder

Hazards associated with ampoules of powder include particle contamination. This is either from the incomplete dissolving of the powder in the diluent, or, when glass ampoules are used, from shards of glass (Dougherty 2002).

(1) Check the ampoule and tap it gently to ensure all the powder is at the bottom.

(2) Cover the top with an alcohol swab and snap it open away from the practitioner. Some ampoules are marked at the neck on the weak area designed to fracture under pressure. Some may require filing. In both instances open with the mark or filed area facing away from the practitioner.

(3) Using a 23 gauge needle (blue), introduce the diluent gently down the side of the ampoule to wet the powder before it is shaken (as above).

(4) Shake the ampoule gently.

(5) Check that the powder is dissolved and that the solution is clear and free from particles.

(6) Aspirate the required volume of the solution with the syringe and 23 gauge (blue) or smaller needle.

(7) Expel the air as described above.

(8) Change the needle for a 25 gauge needle (orange) or other needle-less device for administration of the drug.

(9) Discard used needles into a sharps container.

Preparing ampoules of fluid

Hazards associated with ampoules of fluid include particle contamination from shards of glass when glass ampoules are opened.

(1) Check the ampoule to ensure the fluid is clear and no particles are present.

(2) Tap it gently to ensure all the fluid is at the bottom.

(3) Cover the top with an alcohol swab and snap it open away from the practitioner using the marked weak spot or a file if necessary.

(4) Using a 23 gauge (blue) needle or smaller, aspirate the required volume from the ampoule.

(5) Check the fluid for glass fragments and discard if present.

(6) Aspirate the required volume from the ampoule with the 23 gauge needle (blue) and continue as described above.

Adding drugs to containers of fluid

When adding drugs to containers of fluids or other drug solutions it is imperative to ensure the compatibility of the drug with the fluid it is being added to. Interactions between drugs and solutions may result in a toxic solution or inactivate the therapeutic nature of the drug. Incompatible drug mixtures are not always obvious, with cloudiness or precipitate. Use must be made of drug data sheets, the most recent edition of the *British National Formulary* (BNF), local policy and pharmacists, particularly if there is any uncertainty. Practitioners must be satisfied that pH, concentration and stability of the mixture over time and in the local environment (temperature and light) will all be acceptable. They must also be aware of potential

Table 4.1 Solutions to which drugs must not be added (Dougherty & Lamb 1999, Weinstein 2001)

Blood
Blood products including albumin
Mannitol
Sodium bicarbonate
Dextrans
Parenteral nutrition (except when unavoidable)
Lipid emulsions
Amino acid solutions
Solutions containing other drugs unless their compatibility is
    established, for example cefuroxime and metronidazole IV are
    compatible

---

reactions the patient may experience and how to manage them. There are particular fluids and solutions to which drugs *must not* be added (see Table 4.1).

When drugs are added to containers, or the burette in a burette administration set, the container must be clearly labelled with the following information as a minimum:

- the drug added;
- the dose added;
- the date and time of its addition;
- the signature of the practitioner who added it.

Preparing the infusion with the drug in a container of fluid

Having confirmed the safety of the drug/fluid infusion, assemble all the equipment, fluids and prepared drug as previously described, checking that all the equipment is intact and sterile. Drugs should only be mixed with solutions immediately prior to their use, to reduce the risk of degradation of the drug or growth of contaminating micro-organisms.

(1) Check the prescription.
(2) Lay the container of fluid flat, on a clean surface.
(3) Thoroughly clean the injection port with an alcohol swab and let it dry.

(4) Inject the drug into the bag using a 23 or 25 gauge (blue or orange) needle to enable to the port to re-seal.
(5) Thoroughly mix the container to evenly distribute the drug in the solution.
(6) Check for cloudiness or particles and do not use if present.
(7) Label the container.
(8) Discard waste appropriately.
(9) Prepare to attach the infusion to the patient.
(10) Document the addition of the drug to the fluid appropriately and its subsequent administration to the patient.

Preparing the infusion with the drug in a burette at the bedside

Commence as described above.

(1) Check the prescription and the patient's identity.
(2) Remove bandages over the venous access site.
(3) Ensure the venous access site is clean and not inflamed or showing signs of infiltration.
(4) Clean the injection port of the burette with an alcohol swab and allow it to dry.
(5) Switch off the infusion to the patient.
(6) Fill the burette with the required volume of fluid from the container.
(7) Inject the drug through the injection port.
(8) Mix the drug with the fluid in the burette thoroughly.
(9) Check the mixture for cloudiness or particles – do not use if present.
(10) Label the burette.
(11) Commence the infusion at the required rate.
(12) Ask the patient to report any pain at the site or other unusual sensations indicative of a reaction.
(13) Discard waste into the appropriate container.
(14) Document the administration of the drug and the fluid as indicated.

(15) When complete, recommence the original infusion through the burette.

Preparing drugs for syringe drivers and pumps

When preparing drugs to be administered through a syringe driver or pump, it is important that the infusion is prepared immediately before use. This is to avoid errors that arise from infusions being set up by a practitioner who did not prepare the infusion, or with an infusion intended for another patient.

In addition, interaction of the drug with the plastic syringe and extension tubing or administration set may result in reduction of the active component of the drug infusion, as described in Table 3.1. This includes insulin and glyceryl trinitrate (GTN) infusions. For this reason infusions should be used as soon as they are drawn up and changed every 24 hours.

To prepare a syringe or bag for infusion the drug the drug should be prepared and reconstituted, if necessary, as previously described.

(1) Check the dose and volume to be administered in a 24-hour period. If this is not a fixed rate, for example, an infusion of insulin titrated to hourly blood glucose measurements, an estimate should be made of the volume to be used in 24 hours. It is preferable to change the syringe or bag within that time rather than waste excess or risk running the infusion longer than 24 hours.

(2) Check the volume in which the dose of the drug is to be administered. This should be prescribed and should take into account the patient's fluid balance. In titrated infusions the dose of drug prescribed per hour should, where possible, equate with whole millilitres of fluid so as to facilitate adjusting delivery rates on the pump. For example, an insulin infusion should contain 50 units in a total volume of 50 ml of (0.9% sodium chloride and insulin) to make 1 unit per 1 ml. Thus when 3 units per hour are required the rate of the infusion is 3 ml/hour.

Alternatively, 100 units of insulin could be made up to 50 ml with 0.9% sodium chloride and then for a 3 unit per hour dose the rate of the pump would be 1.5 ml/hour. In this case, the infusion would comprise 1 ml insulin (100 units/ml) and 49 ml 0.9% sodium chloride to total 50 ml. The volume of the infusion comprises the diluent *and* the volume of the drug.

(3) Ensure that the diluent is compatible with the drug.

(4) Using a 23 gauge needle (blue) for glass ampoules or a 21 gauge needle (green) for plastic ampoules, if not a needle-less system, draw up the diluent into the infusion pump syringe.

(5) Expel air carefully into a used ampoule until the correct volume for the infusion is present in the syringe.

(6) Remove the needle.

(7) Withdraw the plunger to make space in the barrel of the syringe with the diluent if using a syringe driver for infusion.

(8) Gently add the correct dose of the drug to the syringe or infusion bag using a separate syringe and needle, and ensure the drug is thoroughly mixed by gently inverting the barrel of the syringe or the bag numerous times. Avoid energetic mixing, as this will cause the mixture to develop air bubbles, and could spray it into the environment from a syringe.

(9) Add the extension or administration set required. For syringe driver infusions, with the syringe tip uppermost, expel the air from the syringe and the extension set.

(10) Label the syringe or bag appropriately.

(11) Prepare to attach the infusion to the patient and set up the syringe driver or pump (see the section on Pumps p 132).

(12) Document the preparation of the infusion and its commencement.

ADMINISTERING DRUGS INTRAVENOUSLY

There are three methods by which drugs may be given intravenously, depending on the patient's treatment and the drug involved. The time in which optimum serum levels are achieved for maximum effect and the drug's toxicity will affect the choice of method.

(1) Direct bolus injection – when peak levels are required as with most antibiotics, or in emergency situations as with adrenaline (epinephrine).
(2) Intermittent infusion – when peak levels are required but a larger volume of dilution is required than possible for a bolus injection.
(3) Continuous infusion – when constant serum levels of a drug are needed for therapeutic effect (Dougherty 2002).

All of the above may be undertaken with or without an existing infusion of compatible fluid in situ, though it is preferable to run continuous drug infusions alone.

Preparing the patient

Prior to administering intravenous drugs to a patient, the aims and procedure should be explained to them in detail. They should understand the need for the therapy, its frequency, its effects and possible side effects, as with any other drug they might take independently. Explaining how the drug will be given may go some way to avoiding needle phobia, if this is a problem. Patients experience less anxiety and stress if they are informed about their treatment and the expected actions and outcomes.

Speed of drug administration

Care must be taken when administering drugs intravenously to avoid causing 'speed-shock'. This arises when a sudden injection of a drug floods the major organs and a toxic reaction occurs. The symptoms are similar to anaphylaxis, including sudden hypotension, tachycardia, collapse and possible cardiac arrest (Sani 1999).

Drug manufacturers provide information about intravenous drug administration and many hospitals have information files for commonly administered intravenous drugs. A pharmacist should be consulted if there is any doubt. The guidance provided should be adhered to. If no information is available, a drug should be administered over three to ten minutes as a minimum if a bolus injection, longer for an intermittent infusion.

In some situations drugs are given rapidly intravenously. These are usually critical situations, including induction of anaesthetic or cardiac arrest, when the drugs in question need to be introduced rapidly to have an effect, and the patient's airway is, or can be, maintained artificially.

Equipment

All the equipment used in setting up intravenous infusions must be sterile and an aseptic technique used in their handling. Any administration set, tubing, stopcock, syringe or injection bung connected to a cannula or administration system must be *luer-locked* in order to avoid inadvertent disconnection, the potential for haemorrhage or air embolism and contamination of the IV system.

Bolus injection without another infusion

This procedure is used for the administration of a drug directly into a venous access device, usually using a syringe and needle or a syringe and needle-less system, through an injectable bung on the device. As described in Chapter 3, the port on top of peripheral cannulae should not be used if at all possible. This is due to their wide aperture and the difficulty in cleaning the cavity, both of which significantly increase the risk of infection and particle infusion. In addition, it is difficult to regulate the rate at which the drug is injected, due to the one-way valve in the port.

(1) The prescription, drug and patient must be checked as previously detailed.

(2) When the drug is prepared for injection, a syringe of 10–20 ml 0.9% sodium chloride should also be prepared for flushing the device before and after the drug injection. In the case of a central catheter used once daily or less frequently, the catheter may require flushing with heparinised saline after the drug is given – local policy should be checked for guidance.

(3) Wash and dry hands thoroughly.

(4) Take the prescription and all the equipment, including a sterile towel, to the patient in a clean tray.

(5) Check the patient's identity and that the drug has not already been given.

(6) Remove the bandages or covering from the device, if present.

(7) Check the insertion site and vein for inflammation or oedema; do not continue if either is present.

(8) Wash hands or rub with alcohol rub.

(9) Place sterile towel under the patient's arm or the device.

(10) Clean the injectable bung thoroughly with alcohol and let it dry naturally.

(11) Flush the device gently using the 0.9% sodium chloride and a 25 gauge (orange) or 23-gauge needle (blue) if using a re-sealing injectable bung to check the device and vein are patent. Observe the insertion site throughout the administration procedure to detect infiltration or reaction early.

(12) Gently administer the drug, using needles as indicated above. (NB a 25 gauge needle (orange) will enable slower administration of the drug.) The rate at which the drug should be given will be dependent on the drug and its toxicity. Data sheets must be consulted prior to administration. For example, a prescription of gentamicin 120 mg three times a day, IV, will require a bolus injection of 120 mg in 3 ml over 3 minutes. That is, a millilitre per

minute. This is due to the ototoxicity of gentamicin. Given faster, the drug may damage the patient's eighth cranial nerve and their hearing and balance.

(13) When the drug infusion is complete, flush the device with 0.9% sodium chloride again to clear the drug from the device and prevent later interactions with incompatible substances.

(14) If more than one drug is being given in a bolus injection, flush the device between each drug and after the last drug. Use a push-stop technique and end with positive pressure to keep the device patent.

(15) Stop the injection if the patient complains of pain or there is resistance to the injection.

(16) Apply a covering dressing or bandage as required.

(17) Ensure the patient is comfortable.

(18) Document the administration of the drug(s).

(19) Discard sharps and waste appropriately.

(20) Wash and dry hands thoroughly.

Box 4.1 Example of administering a bolus IV injection without another infusion

A patient is prescribed a single dose of 600 mg benzylpenicillin IV. They have a peripheral cannula in situ. The drug is prepared in addition to two 5 ml syringes of sodium chloride. The patient's identity, prescription and allergies are checked – he has none he knows of. The cannula site is checked and appears healthy. The cannula has an injection bung attached and this is injected with a syringe of saline attached to a 25 gauge needle (orange). The cannula is easily flushed and the patient denies any discomfort. The benzylpenicillin, reconstituted in 10 ml water for injection, is similarly injected over a period of three minutes. Again, the patient denies any discomfort. The cannula is then flushed again using sodium chloride injection. The flush is delivered in a stop/start manner and the needle withdrawn from the bung whilst a positive pressure is kept on the syringe plunger to prevent obstruction of the cannula with a backflow of blood. The drug administration is recorded on the patient's drug chart.

Bolus injection with an existing infusion

When an infusion is in progress it is possible to administer a compatible drug through the same device. It is important to check the compatibility of the drug with the infusion fluid before commencing. Dilution of the drug with the infusion can help avoid venous irritation (Dougherty 2002).

(1) Prepare the equipment and the patient, as described before.
(2) Check the device insertion site and vein as before, even though the device itself is not being used for the injection; do not proceed if inflammation or oedema is present.
(3) Clean the injection site on the administration set thoroughly with an alcohol swab and allow to dry.
(4) If the patient's infusion is compatible with the drug, it may be used to dilute the drug during its administration.
   • Open the roller clamp on the administration set and check the infusion runs freely. Regulate the rate to drip more quickly.
   • Inject the drug into the set and check that the injection does not slow the drip rate of the infusion. This way the drug is flowing into the vein with the infusion, rather than up into the administration set. Give the drug slowly over the recommended time.
   • Observe the insertion site of the device throughout the injection.
   • If more than one drug is to be given and all are compatible, the administration set should be flushed through by opening the roller clamp to let the infusion run freely between each drug and after the last one is completed.
(5) Check the patient is comfortable.
(6) Finish the procedure as described before.
   • If the infusion in situ is not compatible with the drug, the administration set should be turned off and flushed with 0.9% sodium chloride to clear the administration set before administering the drug.

- This should be repeated between each drug and after the last one to avoid interaction between incompatible substances.
- If the patient is fluid restricted, do not use the technique of running the infusion more quickly. Turn the infusion off and use 5 ml of 0.9% sodium chloride to flush the set before and after giving the drug.

Box 4.2 Example of administering a bolus IV injection with an existing infusion

A prescription for hydrocortisone, 100 mg, six hourly, IV, is written for a patient with an exacerbation of ulcerative colitis. The patient is receiving a continuous infusion of 0.9% sodium chloride at a rate of 1 L in eight hours. 100 mg hydrocortisone is reconstituted in 2 ml of water for injection, and is compatible with 0.9% sodium chloride. The patient's infusion and IV site are checked, as is the prescription and the patient's identity. The infusion rate is increased slightly to dilute the drug. The drug is administered into the administration set of the 0.9% sodium chloride infusion by injection, slowly, over several minutes. At the same time the rate of the drip is watched to ensure it is not slowed by the pressure of the injection. This achieves a measured rate of infusion and additional dilution of the drug. When the drug is given, the infusion rate is further increased to flush the administration set and IV device and then regulated to the prescribed rate.

Intermittent drug infusion without an existing infusion

When a patient needs to be given an intravenous drug intermittently to achieve peak serum levels, but the drug requires dilution to avoid toxic effects, it is given in an infusion of compatible fluid.

(1) Prepare the patient to receive the infusion and prepare the infusion as described previously with the drug added to an infusion of compatible fluid in an appropriate volume. Prepare a 10 ml syringe of 0.9% sodium chloride for flushing the device before the infusion.

(2)   Check the prescription, the drug and the infusion fluid are correct.

(3)   Wash and dry hands thoroughly.

(4)   Take the prescription and all the equipment, including a sterile towel, to the patient in a clean tray.

(5)   Check the patient's identity and that the drug has not already been given.

(6)   Remove the bandages or covering from the device, if present.

(7)   Check the insertion site and vein for redness, oedema or signs of infiltration; do not proceed if present.

(8)   Wash hands or rub with alcohol rub.

(9)   Place sterile towel under the patient's arm or the device.

(10) Clean the injectable bung thoroughly with alcohol and let it dry naturally.

(11) Flush the device gently using the 0.9% sodium chloride and a 25 gauge (orange) or 23 gauge (blue) needle if using a re-sealing injectable bung, to check the device and vein are patent. Do not proceed if there is any doubt.

(12) Observe the insertion site.

(13) Connect the infusion to the device and commence the infusion at the required rate.

(14) Check the patient is comfortable and ask them to report any pain at the insertion site, or symptoms of reaction, including difficulty breathing, feeling faint or developing an itching rash.

(15) Secure the infusion administration set so that it does not put tension on the device and cause phlebitis.

(16) Only re-apply the bandage if the device will be at risk from the patient's movement during the infusion, and/or the infusion will run for longer than 30 minutes.

(17) Observe the insertion site intermittently throughout the administration procedure to detect infiltration or reaction early.

(18) When the infusion is complete take a further 10 ml syringe of 0.9% sodium chloride and sterile injectable bung to the patient.

(19) Wash and dry hands thoroughly.

(20) Disconnect the infusion and attach the sterile injectable bung or similar device. The infusion bag and administration set must be discarded.

(21) Flush the cannula with the 0.9% sodium chloride injecting through the bung with a 25 gauge (orange) or 23 gauge (blue) needle to clear the drug from the device. Use a push-stop technique and end with positive pressure to keep the device patent.

(22) Apply a covering dressing or bandage as required.

(23) Ensure the patient is comfortable.

(24) Document the administration of the drug and infusion volume.

(25) Discard sharps and waste appropriately.

(26) Wash and dry hands thoroughly.

Box 4.3 Example of administering an intermittent drug infusion without an existing infusion

A patient being treated with erythromycin 500 mg six hourly, IV, will have an infusion prepared with 500 mg erythromycin reconstituted in 10 ml of water for injection. The drug will then be added to a minimum of 100 ml of 0.9% sodium chloride and infused over 20–60 minutes (BNF 2003). The IV device will be flushed to check its patency before the infusion is attached and commenced, as it will be after the infusion is completed. The infusion set is discarded after each dose, unless it is left connected to the patient's IV device, in which case it is changed every 24 hours.

Intermittent drug infusion with an existing fluid infusion

Adapted administration sets for attaching two infusions to the same device are available and can be useful for patients who are dependent on continuous infusions of fluid and require regular intermittent drug infusions. Alternatively, extension sets and three-way stopcocks or switching devices may be used. As previously stated, the fewer additions made to infusion sets the less likely the risk of contamination from the connections and the manipulation of the equipment, particularly three-way taps. However, where it is necessary to use a three-way tap for a peripheral cannula, it should *never* be directly attached to the cannula. Manipulating the three-way tap at the connection to the cannula will cause two problems.

(1) A significantly higher risk of contamination due to the inherently unhygienic nature of three-way taps, and the proximity of the practitioner's hands to the insertion site every time the tap is turned.
(2) Phlebitis is highly likely to occur, as the cannula will rub against the intima of the vein every time the tap is turned, even if it is well secured.

If a three-way tap must be used, these risks can be reduced by adding an extension set to the cannula, adding the three-way tap to the end of the extension set, connecting the fluid infusion to the three-way tap and intermittently using the side tap of the three-way tap through which to administer the drug infusion. The three-way tap should be secured to the patient's arm, and protected from contamination by the skin flora with a sterile, low-linting piece of gauze (see Fig 4.3). The device may then be bandaged as required. This way the repeated manipulations of the tap will not be near the device to risk contamination, or cause movement of the device in the vein.

(1) Prepare the patient and the equipment, as described earlier.
(2) Check the prescription, the drug and the infusion fluid are correct.
(3) Wash and dry hands thoroughly.
(4) Take the prescription and all the equipment to the patient in a clean tray.

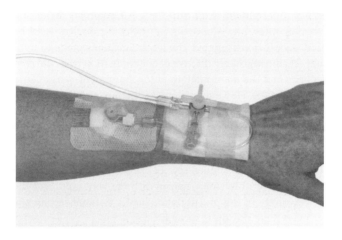

Fig. 4.3 Using a three-way tap on a peripheral cannula

(5) Check the patient's identity and that the drug has not already been given.

(6) Check the device insertion site and vein as before, even though the device is not being used for the injection; do not proceed if there is oedema or inflammation.

(7) Open the roller clamp on the administration set and check the infusion runs freely, then turn off the infusion.

(8) Uncover and clean the port on the administration set thoroughly with an alcohol swab and allow to dry.

(9) If the drug is not compatible with the fluid infusion, flush the extension set and cannula with 10 ml 0.9% sodium chloride through the side arm of the three-way tap to clear the tubing.

(10) Connect the drug infusion to the side arm of the three-way tap and turn the tap so that the fluid infusion is off and the drug infusion will run into the patient's cannula.

(11) Adjust the rate of the drug infusion as required.

(12) Only re-apply the bandage if the device will be at risk from the patient's movement during the infusion, and/or the infusion will run for longer than 30 minutes.

(13) Observe the insertion site of the device intermittently throughout the injection.

(14) Wash and dry hands thoroughly before handling the three-way tap.

(15) When the infusion is complete, turn the three-way tap off to the drug infusion. Flush the tubing with 0.9% sodium chloride again if required.

(16) Turn the three-way tap so that the fluid infusion can be recommenced, and adjust its drip rate appropriately.

(17) Disconnect and discard the infusion set, if indicated, and attach the sterile bung or similar device. It may be possible to leave the drug infusion set attached for the next dose, changing it every 24 hours, as with the specially adapted administration sets (Nichol 1999).

(18) Apply a covering dressing or bandage as required.

(19) Ensure the patient is comfortable.

(20) Document the administration of the drug and infusion volume.

(21) Discard sharps and waste appropriately.

(22) Wash and dry hands thoroughly.

Box 4.4 Example of administering an intermittent drug infusion with an existing infusion

An example of this type of IV therapy would be that for a patient who is dependent on a crystalloid infusion for hydration (see Table 5.1) and requires metronidazole 500 mg (prepared in 100 ml), eight hourly, IV. Provided the infusion fluid is compatible with the metronidazole, a specially adapted administration set with two infusion 'arms' may be used, or an extension set and three-way tap as described above. The administration set for the drug must be changed every 24 hours.

Continuous drug infusion without another infusion

When a patient's therapy requires a constant, specific level of a drug in the blood, a continuous drug infusion is used. This may be achieved either in a syringe or container with an infusion pump, or for a slow infusion by a manually regulated administration set. It is rare to infuse IV drugs continuously without a pump as the risk of fluctuating levels is too great and in contradiction to the intentions of the treatment.

The patient should be prepared for having the infusion, paying particular attention to ensuring their understanding of what the drug is for and what effects it may have, when this is possible. The patient needs to understand what the early signs of side effects might be and to report these early. If, for example, monitoring the patient's blood sugar, or blood pressure and pulse is required more frequently whilst the infusion is in progress, they should be made aware of this at the start.

(1) When preparing a drug for continuous infusion, steps need to be taken to prepare the drug in the appropriate diluent and container as described earlier.

(2) Clearly label the container the drug is added to, so that its name and the dose per ml can be easily seen at all times.

(3) Take the steps described previously to set up the infusion.

(4) Re-bandage the patient's arm if indicated, but remember to check the insertion site regularly (at least three times a day).

(5) Change the entire administration equipment every 24 hours, even if the infusion is not complete. This will avoid administering a less active solution of the drug, or a solution into which plasticiser from the administration tubing has leached.

(6) If another drug is prescribed for intravenous administration and the infusion is attached to the only site of access, consider adding a three-way tap and extension tube to the cannula, or a three-way tap to the end of the catheter and

giving the drug through it. Ensure that the extension set is flushed completely with 0.9% sodium chloride before and after the drug is given and the infusion recommenced.

(7) Document the administration of the drug clearly, as well as the patient's response to it.

Box 4.5 Example of administering a continuous drug infusion without an existing infusion

When suffering acute angina a patient requires a glyceryl trinitrate (GTN) infusion, run at 100 micrograms per minute. The drug is dispensed in ampoules of 5 or 10 ml, in a concentration of 5 mg/ml. The infusion is prepared by drawing up one ampoule of 10 ml, equivalent to 50 mg (10×5 mg/ml) and diluting it with 40 ml of 0.9% sodium chloride solution to make a solution of 50 mg in 50 ml, that is a concentration of 1 mg/1 ml. Once the prescription, the patient and the device patency are checked, the infusion is set up with a syringe pump and the appropriately labelled syringe, and the extension tubing is luer-locked onto the patient's cannula. To deliver 100 micrograms per minute the rate is set at 6 ml per hour. This is calculated as follows

$$\text{ml/hr} = \frac{\text{micrograms/minute} \times 60 \text{ (minutes per hour)}}{\text{micrograms/ml (concentration of the infusion)}}$$

$$\text{ml/hr} = \frac{100 \text{ micrograms} \times 60}{1000 \text{ micrograms/ml}}$$

$$\text{ml/hr} = \frac{6000}{1000}$$

$$\text{ml/hr} = 6$$

(See Chapter 6 for more about calculations)

Continuous drug infusion with an existing fluid infusion

It is always preferable for drug infusions to be administered singly into separate devices to avoid the risks of incompatibility. When a patient has an infusion running and an additional, continuous infusion is required, it is preferable for the drug infusion to have its own venous access for administration, even if the drug and the fluid are compatible. The principal danger of running two infusions into one device is that the constant flow of either into the patient's vein cannot be guaranteed or monitored. If there is an obstruction of flow anywhere in the system, the fluids being infused will take the path of least resistance. If the obstruction is then released, flow will resume, but it may be sudden and could result in an accidental bolus of a drug being given. Thus the prescribed continuous rate of administration will not be achieved and could be dangerous for the patient. Any opiate, sedative or patient-controlled analgesia (PCA) infusion must always have dedicated IV access for this reason.

Box 4.6 Example of the potential difficulties of administering a continuous drug infusion with an existing infusion

A patient with a continuous infusion of dextrose saline has an infusion of morphine running for pain relief. The practitioner caring for the patient notes that the peripheral cannula is over the patient's wrist joint and the infusion of fluid is not running, though the morphine infusion appears to be continuing. The patient is not as comfortable as she was an hour ago. On securing the IV device and reminding the patient to keep her wrist straight, the infusion runs freely again. Within a few minutes the patient is pain-free but somewhat drowsy. With the resistance to flow into the vein caused by the device being flexed, the morphine infusion (which was under higher pressure than the fluid infusion) was pumped up the fluid infusion administration set. When the resistance was released, an uncontrolled bolus dose of morphine was administered to the patient via the infusion administration set in a matter of seconds.

Only when it really is not possible to have dedicated venous access for a drug infusion and a compatible fluid infusion is also required, can one device be used for both. Careful consideration must be given to monitoring the infusions' flow, the effect of the drug on the patient, and the site of the device to ensure that both infusions are running consistently as prescribed and that the device remains patent.

(1) The infusions should be prepared as previously detailed.
(2) The patient should be prepared for the infusions as previously described.
(3) The infusions should be connected to the device using extension tubing and a three-way tap or similar device such as a 'Y' connector which enables both infusions to run concurrently or singly (each can be switched off separately). It is vital that manipulations are undertaken at a distance from a peripheral cannula, as described earlier, when giving intermittent drug infusions with continuous fluid infusions.
(4) The drug infusion must be clearly labelled in a manner that is visible at all times.
(5) All the administration tubing should be changed every 24 hours, as described above, and the shortest length to allow movement used.
(6) The infusion rates of the drug and the fluid must be monitored regularly to ensure their correct rate of flow.
(7) The device and insertion site must be regularly checked for patency and signs of inflammation or oedema.
(8) Infusions should be stopped at the earliest signs of problems with flow or the insertion site or the patient's condition.
(9) Document the administration of the drug and the fluid clearly, as well as the patient's response to it.

ADMINISTERING DRUGS THROUGH MULTIPLE LUMEN CENTRAL CATHETERS

The principles for preparing drugs and infusions for administration described earlier, should also be followed when using CVADs. Catheters with more than one lumen allow the administration of incompatible drugs and infusions simultaneously. Devices for short-term use have separate exit points (Fig. 3.11)

> **Box 4.7** Example of administering a continuous drug infusion
> with an existing infusion
>
> A patient with a suspected thrombosis and dehydration is
> prescribed 1 litre 0.9% sodium chloride over 12 hours (repeated),
> and heparin, 25 000 units in 25 ml 0.9% sodium chloride at 1 ml
> per hour. This patient has a single peripheral cannula in situ and
> poor peripheral veins due to previous IV therapy. The infusions
> are prepared, the heparin having been drawn up in a 50 ml luer
> connection syringe for infusion in a syringe driver pump. An
> extension tube is attached to the patient's cannula that has been
> checked for patency and is free flowing. The heparin syringe has
> an extension tube connected to it and this is luer-locked onto a
> three-way tap. The 0.9% sodium chloride infusion is also
> connected to the three-way tap and this in turn is connected to
> the extension tube on the patient's cannula. For security, the
> tubing between the tap and the cannula is secured to the
> patient's arm with a piece of sterile gauze to protect it from
> colonisation by skin organisms. When the infusions are
> connected the tap is turned so that both infusions flow into the
> patient's vein. The pump rate is set as prescribed and the fluid
> infusion commenced. The rates of both are monitored hourly,
> checking that the fluid infusion drip rate does not slow. This
> might indicate an occlusion developing in the cannula or
> elsewhere in the administration equipment and could indicate
> inaccurate delivery of the heparin.

to prevent mixing of infusions at the end of the catheter in the
vein or right atrium. Principles of compatibility still apply to
the administration of drugs and infusions down each lumen.

If a catheter with multiple lumens is being used to measure
a patient's CVP, it is preferable to measure the CVP using the
distal lumen. This most accurately represents CVP, with 'back-
pressure' of blood on the end of the catheter as opposed to that
of blood flowing past an exit point on the side of the catheter,
as the proximal and middle lumens do. The same lumen must
always be used for comparable readings.

It is not advisable to use the lumen through which CVP
measurements are taken for infusions other than crystalloid

infusions. If drug infusions are also connected, the residual drug in the tubing and the lumen of the catheter will not be administered smoothly. Infusions will need to be stopped for measurements to be taken and the drug in the tubing could be delivered in a bolus when the tubing is primed for the reading, or as the pressure level falls.

INFUSION BY GRAVITY

Running an infusion using a simple administration set and gravity is familiar to all health care professionals and is suitable for numerous patients having IV therapy. However, it is important to remember that infusions which run by gravity may not be delivered accurately or consistently, and that a number of factors will affect the rate of flow.

(1) Type of fluid
 • more viscous fluid flows more slowly;
 • substances irritant to the vein cause venous spasm and slow infusion.
(2) Temperature of the fluid
 • cold fluids cause venous spasm, slowing the infusion – a warm compress will help.
(3) Height of the container in comparison to the patient
 • the higher the container the greater the force of gravity and the rate of flow.
(4) Administration set and equipment (extension tubing, stopcocks).
(5) Roller clamp on the administration set
 • this can become loose and allow faster flow, or alter the tubing shape and affect flow;
 • may be interfered with and flow altered.
(6) Type and size of IV device
 • the larger the diameter of the device, the faster the flow.
(7) Location of IV device
 • when the device is placed over a joint, flexion of the joint may kink it and flow rate will slow or stop;

- if the end of the device is against the wall of the vein or a valve, flow rate is reduced.

(8) Occlusion of the device or tubing (partial or complete)
- with clot or fibrin in the lumen of the device the flow is slower or stops;
- kinking of the tubing reduces flow.

(9) Size and condition of the vein
- small or damaged veins will have a lower flow rate.

Practitioners must be vigilant in monitoring flow rates of infusions by gravity. This includes calculating the correct rate of flow for the infusion according to the set used (see Chapter 6), monitoring the approximate rate of infusion regularly, as well as checking that the IV site and administration equipment are not obstructed (Weinstein 2001).

It is important to note that the height of the infusion above the patient affects the rate of flow. If the patient moves and the distance between the patient's device and the container for the infusion changes, so will the rate of flow. For example, a patient who has had an infusion commenced whilst sitting in a chair, is later helped back to bed. The bed is lowered and leaves the patient approximately 60 cm lower than when he was in the chair. If the infusion roller clamp is not re-adjusted to regulate the infusion rate to that prescribed, the infusion will run more quickly than originally intended. Similarly, if the patient is ambulant and adjusts the height of the infusion to get through doorways, but does not return the drip stand to the former height, the infusion rate will slow down. This emphasises the need for continual observation by the practitioner responsible for the patient's care.

PUMPS

Intravenous therapy has developed considerably over the last three decades and this has been partly due to the development of electronic appliances or mechanical infusion devices that can control the rate of flow of an infusion. Some of the appliances used in IV therapy have a pumping action, others function differently, as will be described in Table 4.2, but for easy reference these appliances will be collectively referred to here as 'pumps'.

Critically ill patients, including those at particular risk from inaccurate infusion (the very young, the elderly, and highly dependent patients in a critical condition or requiring multiple therapies) have benefited most from technological advances in infusion pumps. Unlike relying on gravity for the infusion of a drug or fluids, pumps accurately regulate the rate of flow of fluid into the patient, administering a constant volume (or dose) over a set period of time. This has improved the safety of IV therapy considerably.

When to use a pump

Practitioners need to be familiar with the equipment available to them in order to make appropriate choices for their patients. When a patient requires a specific infusion at a specific rate, and over- or under-infusion would present a risk to the patient, a pump should be used to deliver the infusion.

The type of pump to be used will depend on:

- the volume and rate of infusion;
- the accuracy required;
- the alarms required and their sensitivity;
- the type of drug or fluid being infused (e.g. viscosity);
- the patient's need (e.g. critically ill, neonate);
- their mobility;
- how easy the pump is to use;
- how often it will need adjustment and by whom (Dolan 1999).

Where the patient is likely to require the device for longer than a few days, and if they are able to participate in decision-making about their care, it is preferable to involve them in the choice of appliance if possible.

> **Box 4.8** Pump or gravity?
>
> When there is a choice among using a pump, gravity and a basic administration set to infuse fluid (that is, for patients who are not critically ill or receiving drugs or potentially toxic fluids), the practitioner must consider whether the advantages of using the pump outweigh the risks. It is advantageous to have fluids infuse more accurately, but pumps are not a substitute for monitoring patients' infusions, the site of the IV device or the effect of the infusion on the patient. Alarms can be distressing to patients and staff, and the pressure at which fluids are pumped could be high and potentially damaging, to the vein, or if infiltration occurs, or if a bolus is infused after an occlusion is released.

Knowledge and accountability

As with any other aspect of practice, it is important to stress that knowledge of procedure and, here, the equipment being used, is imperative. Ignorance about the operating of an appliance is no excuse should it be found to have administered the wrong volume in a given time and caused harm to the patient. Training in the specific types of pump in use in a clinical area or care service is vital and should be available to new staff and when new equipment is purchased. Practitioners should then have the opportunity to practise using the appliances with supervision, and become competent in handling them so that they can use the pumps safely.

Before using a pump, practitioners must know:

- how to set up the device appropriately;
- how it should work;
- what monitoring is required to check its function;
- what dedicated equipment should be used with the pump (e.g. administration sets);
- how to recognise malfunction;
- what to do in the event of an adverse incident involving the pump (Glenister 2001).

Types of infusion pump

Features of infusion pumps include:

- accuracy of flow;
- volume of flow rates;
- volume to be infused (VTBI) setting; the pump will stop and alarm when the set volume has been infused;
- keep vein open (KVO) setting; this rate infuses at a slow rate (depending on the pump) until an infusion can be stopped or changed;
- alarms for
  - air in the line;
  - occlusion; sensors detect occlusions in the tubing above (upstream) or below (downstream) the pump; pressure sensitivity can be selected in some models for occlusions in the line between the pump and the patient's infusion device. The time taken for the alarm to sound after the occlusion begins depends on the rate of flow and the pressure sensitivity the pump is set to. When the alarm starts, the pressure in the tubing will be raised, as the fluid will have built up under pressure in order for the alarm to sound. Care must be taken when freeing the occlusion to avoid a bolus of the infusion running straight into the vein. This could mean an overdose and damage the patient's vein.

Infusion pumps have been classified by the Medical and Healthcare products Regulatory Agency into three groups according to their features and suitability for specific uses.

(1) Neonatal – those with the highest accuracy and lowest volume incremental settings (0.1 ml), high sensitivity and short alarm delay times, low bolus infusion on release of occlusion, automatic switching from mains to battery power.

(2) High risk – usually used for drug administration, these pumps have high accuracy, high sensitivity and short

alarm delay times, low bolus infusion volume and automatic mains to battery changeover.

(3) Low risk – these pumps are used for fluid and drug infusions where less accuracy is essential (such as parenteral nutrition or antibiotics), alarms are less sensitive and flow may be less accurate.

With developments in medical technology a large range of infusion appliances are now manufactured. For clarification these can all be divided into four main types.

(1) Syringe pumps.
(2) Infusion pumps.
(3) Gravity controllers.
(4) Ambulatory pumps.

The characteristics of more commonly used pumps can be found in Table 4.2.

Using pumps
Any practitioner using a pump for a patient's IV infusion, or looking after a patient with an existing infusion, is accountable for the therapy delivered to the patient whilst in their care. This means that the practitioner must know:

- the indications for use of the particular pump;
- where user instructions are and must be familiar with them;
- how the pump works;
- how to use the pump safely and be competent in this;
- what dedicated equipment the pump requires, if any, and where to get it;
- what the limitations of the pump are;
- how to check that the pump is infusing as programmed;
- how to troubleshoot when the pump does not appear to function;
- what to do if the pump fails, including reporting adverse incidents;
- where to get another pump if required.

Table 4.2 Commonly used pumps (Dolan 1999, Dougherty 2000b, Weinstein 2001)

Pump type	Uses	Features	Advantages	Disadvantages
Syringe NB Use luer-lock syringes to attach to infusion tubing where possible to avoid accidental disconnection.	Syringe infusion pumps	• Fluids and drugs for neonates and children • Drugs for adults	• Accurate • Low volume settings ml/hour • Some have memory of programming and servicing which is useful • Up to 60 ml volume depending on syringe used • Plunger and barrel of syringe must be accurately inserted and clamped for accurate function • Some have locked syringe holders • Mains and battery powered	• Alarm for inaccurate insertion is preferable • Alarm when syringe empty, syringe clamp open alarm, battery low alarm	• Few on newer models (since 1996) • Ensure attached horizontally to promote accuracy and facilitate reading the pump settings, syringe label and volume infused markings.

Table 4.2 *Continued*

Pump type	Uses	Features	Advantages	Disadvantages
Syringe drivers	• Drugs for adults where high accuracy level is not essential	• Hourly or 24 hourly rate • Calibrated in mm/hr or 24 hours • Use smallest syringe possible to improve accuracy • Battery powered only	• Small and lightweight • Do not require dedicated equipment • Cheaper to buy and maintain • Alarm if syringe plunger obstructed	• Minimum functions and alarms • Deliver small volumes intermittently rather than continuous flow • Less accurate • Battery operation only – spare batteries must be available
Patient-controlled analgesia (PCA) pumps	• Infusions of opiates for pain control with prescribed bolus doses on demand • Commonly used for post-operative pain control • Acute and chronic pain control	• Programmed to deliver a 'bolus' dose when hand-held button pressed • Programmed 'lock-out' time prevents 'over-dose'. Boluses cannot be repeated within	• Should be easy to use and involves patients in their pain therapy • Reduce patients' pain and anxiety, increasing recovery rate • Reduce nursing time • Similar advantages	• Expensive to purchase • Continuous infusions seldom used post-operatively and should not be used if there is any possibility of the patient receiving

Infusion pumps

		lock-out time • May have additional background or continuous infusion • History of doses requested and doses given indicates efficacy of pain control or use by patient • Patients need to be shown how to use it • Some have locked syringe holders • Mains and battery powered	and alarms to other syringe pumps • Most use standard syringes and tubing	excessive dose of opiate • Staff in clinical areas must be trained in using these pumps' unique features
Volumetric pumps	• All large volume infusions	• Measure the volume infused against a pre-set volume to be infused; alarm when complete • Some have KVO function • Use a reservoir	• Accurate • Wide range of volume delivery • Air-in-line sensors • End of infusion alarm • Low battery alarm • Some have	• Expensive to buy and use • Need dedicated administration sets • Some are complex to set up, increasing errors

Table 4.2 *Continued*

Pump type	Uses	Features	Advantages	Disadvantages
		cassette with standard volume capacity, or linear peristaltic wave-like motion to push fluid through the administration set • Mains and battery powered	adjustable pressure sensors • Some have secondary infusion mechanism for intermittent infusions, switching back to the original infusion when complete	
Volumetric controllers	• Large volume infusions where accuracy is not critical	• Set in ml/hour • Drop sensor • Ensures no over-infusion • Mains or battery powered	• Easy to use • Sensitive alarms • Low infusion pressure • Less expensive than infusion pumps	• Usually need dedicated sets • Only accurate within 10%
Gravity controllers No mechanical pumping is involved. Constricting the infusion set controls rate of flow in conjunction with the height				

of the infusion (gravity).				
Drip rate controllers	• Large volume infusions where accuracy is not critical	• Drop sensor counts drops per minute • Ensures no over-infusion • Mains or battery powered	• Usually need standard administration sets • Less expensive than volumetric controller	• Drop volume varies with different fluids but drop counter function does not take account of this
Ambulatory pumps Syringe drivers Volumetric	• See above • As above but smaller, portable size • Enables patients to have treatment at home • Cancer chemotherapy • Some have PCA type functions	• Compact, light-weight • Easy to use • Can infuse intermittently or continuously • Small reservoir for small volume infusions • Can be set up for weeks or months of infusion • Audible alarms • Battery powered	• Reliable and durable • Accurate • Continuous administration of drugs can improve treatment outcomes • Use by the patient at home increases their involvement, independence and control	• As commonly used in the community users need a point of contact if problems arise • Expensive

The majority of reported 'incidents' or malfunctions with pumps are due to user error rather than an actual fault with the pump itself (Whyte 2001), the most common error being over-infusion due to the wrong infusion rate being set.

Setting up an infusion

(1) Where possible, prepare the patient for the infusion, explaining the need for the therapy, the rationale for using the equipment, the alarm systems and when to call for help.

(2) Ensure the pump is clean, is in working order and settings are zeroed before setting up the equipment.

(3) Mount the pump correctly on an appropriate, stable stand. Ensure that the pump settings and the administration equipment will be clearly visible in the position it is mounted in. The pump should not be too high on the stand; if the centre of gravity of the pump and stand are too high, they may be unstable and fall over when moved.

If several pumps are in use on the same stand, ensure pumps are balanced on the stand or use more than one stand.

(4) Prepare the infusion using equipment appropriate for the pump.

(5) Ensure all air is removed from the infusion set before setting up the pump.

(6) Calculate the rate of the infusion.

(7) Correctly load the pump with the infusion set, ensuring that the label detailing the contents of the infusion is clearly visible without having to unload the pump. If a syringe pump is being used, ensure the syringe volume markings are also clearly visible without having to unload the pump.

(8) Check the prescription, the patient's identification and the infusion are all correct.

(9) Prepare the patient's IV device for connection to the infusion using a sterile towel and aseptic technique.

(10) When connected, correctly alter the pump settings to the required levels for the patient's infusion.

(11) Commence the infusion, having released in-line clamps on CVADs if required.

(12) Check the rate of the infusion regularly within the first hour to ensure correct functioning of the pump.

(13) Document commencement and rate of delivery of the infusion. For syringe pumps this can be done accurately by recording on a regular basis the volume remaining in the syringe barrel. Estimation of the volume remaining in a larger volume infusion, such as parenteral nutrition, can be undertaken and compared with the volume infused reading on the pump.

Continuing infusions

When practitioners' shifts change and patient care is handed over, including an ongoing infusion, the infusion contents, the pump and the IV device site must be checked by the practitioner taking over the patient's care. It is important to be satisfied that:

- the infusion is as prescribed;
- the infusion is running as prescribed into a patent device;
- the pump settings are correct;
- the pump is functioning.

Ensure the pump is connected to the mains whenever possible, if not solely battery operated. Pumps that run on mains or battery charge the battery when connected to the mains and should be replaced if the battery is low or not charging. Pumps not in use should be connected to the mains to charge the batteries.

Pumps dependent on batteries to function (e.g. syringe drivers) should not use rechargeable batteries, and a store of replacement batteries must be readily available.

Continue to document the delivery of the infusion.

Changing infusions

When an infusion is complete and another is required, the pump should be stopped *and* the infusion should be turned off, or the device occluded to avoid a bolus or free-flow of the fluid being delivered to the patient when the pump is unloaded. A new infusion should be prepared and commenced as described under 'Setting up an infusion'. Completion of the previous infusion should be documented, as should commencement of the new.

Infusion equipment (tubing and administration sets) for drug or parenteral nutrition infusions should be changed every 24 to 48 hours when the infusion is compete (Tait 2000).

Completing an infusion

(1) On completion of an infusion, the pump should be stopped and the infusion set switched off, or the device occluded as described above.
(2) Using aseptic technique, disconnect the infusion.
(3) Flush the patient's IV device with 0.9% sodium chloride solution to clear the device of the infusate.
(4) Cap off the device with a sterile injectable bung (for future flushing) or similar.
(5) Ensure the patient is comfortable.
(6) Document the completion of the infusion.
(7) Remove the pump and infusion equipment and dispose of the infusion set and any remaining infusate appropriately.
(8) Zero the pump settings.
(9) Clean the pump as instructed by the manufacturer (do not use alcohol).
(10) Remove the battery if battery-dependent.
(11) Plug into the mains to charge, if battery and mains operated.

If a pump has malfunctioned, been dropped or otherwise damaged it must be immediately withdrawn from use in a clinical area and sent for repair, with details of the problem which arose. Pumps *must not* be mended by practitioners in the clinical setting, as hidden damage could cause serious malfunction, with lethal implications for a patient. Pumps must be regularly serviced as directed by the manufacturer.

Getting the best out of pumps

Whilst pumps have improved the possibilities for patients' IV therapy dramatically, they are not without their drawbacks, including:

- confusion about operating pumps when complex models are used or numerous different types of pump are used;
- their potential for serious or lethal effects on the patient if correct rates of infusion are not achieved;
- stress to patients and practitioners from alarms and lack of consistent infusion;
- lack of availability of the right pump for the patient, clean and in good working order (Dougherty 2000b).

Most of the difficulties which arise with pumps (and other electronic or mechanical equipment) can be avoided with appropriate planning and organisation of their use in clinical practice.

Purchasing

Most pumps are expensive to buy and maintain, and their widespread use in clinical care means that numerous practitioners and patients are likely to use a pump within its working lifetime. Involvement of clinical staff in decision-making about purchasing will ensure that the day-to-day practicalities of using particular pieces of equipment will be considered.

The use of fewer models of a particular kind of pump, e.g. syringe pump, is important to improve staff knowledge of the device and reduce error. In addition, consideration needs to be given to ongoing costs. When a particular pump requires dedicated infusion equipment it will not be as adaptable or cost-efficient to maintain as one which runs with universally available infusion sets.

Staff training

As already highlighted, practitioners are accountable for their practice and must ensure they have the requisite knowledge to care for patients using the equipment available in their clinical area. Employers are responsible for ensuring that adequate training is provided for practitioners about the equipment available for their use so that patient safety is optimised and the equipment in use is familiar to users. The training must include:

- what the pump is suitable for;
- how to mount the pump on a stand for use;
- how to set up the pump with administration equipment;
- what settings are included on the pump and how to adjust them;
- how to avoid problems, including air in the line or free-flow of infusate;
- how to clean and store the pump;
- how to access manufacturers' instructions;
- practical sessions on setting up and handling the pump, and troubleshooting.

Staff must also be aware of the importance of:

- monitoring infusions and pump function whilst infusions are in progress;
- detecting and reporting adverse incidents;
- removing potentially faulty devices from clinical areas (Glenister 2001).

Teaching programmes should be included as part of orientation programmes, be undertaken when new equipment is purchased before it is presented for use by practitioners, and be accessible in continuous professional development programmes for updating and refreshing practitioners' knowledge. Records of training and education undertaken must be kept.

Maintenance and storage

Electronic equipment must be maintained in clean, safe and working order for use by the next patient. A system for tracking equipment is important in achieving this. It is preferable that electronic equipment be centrally stored so that it is easily retrieved for future use. In this way, significant time is saved in obtaining and maintaining equipment. Devices can be checked in and out of the store, a database of available equipment can be kept, battery/mains pumps can be left connected to the mains whilst not in use to charge batteries, and equipment can be cleaned between uses and repaired and serviced when required. The organisation of the equipment store can include the running of training programmes for new and existing equipment on a repeated basis to maintain practitioners' knowledge of the devices in use.

It is important to remember that a pump is only as good as the person using it, and only when it is well maintained. Pumps need to be appropriately used, set up and operated to fulfil their function. They are not a substitute for assessment and suitable intervention in a patient's care.

DOCUMENTATION

In many centres IV therapy has not been routinely documented, other than keeping a record of fluid balance and the administration of prescribed drugs. However, there is much more information which needs to be recorded than the fluid volume or administration of a drug prescription. This includes:

(1) Siting of devices
   - the type of device;
   - the site of insertion;

- the date and time;
- the name and signature of the practitioner inserting the device.

(2) Disposable equipment use
- the date and time infusion sets, extension tubing, three-way taps, injection caps or other in-line infusion equipment is changed;
- the name and signature of the practitioner changing the equipment.

(3) Administration of IV therapy
- completing the prescription record that the drug has been given;
- recording the volume infused where indicated by the patient's condition;
- recording the progress of the infusion over time – that is, checking the infusion is running as prescribed. Where a pump is used, this must be done to ensure the pump is functioning as set. This will facilitate the early detection of error and reduce the impact on the patient;
- recording the effect of the therapy on the patient at intervals during the treatment (e.g. pain control with PCA infusions, blood pressure measurement with GTN, blood glucose levels with insulin infusions).

(4) Incident reporting
- adverse effects of IV therapy on the patient (e.g. drug reaction or over-infusion);
- recording the infiltration or extravasation of an infusion;
- recording episodes of phlebitis or thrombophlebitis, site sepsis or septicaemia, or other complications of IV therapy;
- recording accidental removal of IV devices;
- recording errors in pump functions or damage incurred to pumps whilst in use.

The purpose of keeping records of this information is to promote:

- professional practice through high standards of care;
- continuity of care;
- communication and dissemination of information about patients' therapy and response;
- keeping an accurate account of the patient's therapy;
- the ability to detect problems early (NMC 2002).

It is also for the purpose of auditing care. For example, using the data generated about the placement of peripheral cannulae, the frequency with which they are re-sited and the incidence of phlebitis could indicate the need for a change in practice where cannulae are changed infrequently and the incidence of phlebitis is high. Guidance about changing equipment to reduce the rate of infection is only useful when it is known how long it is since the equipment was last changed.

Practitioners' clinical areas will have, or will need to develop, methods for accurately recording this information that is most suited to the area of practice. Where care pathways or electronic records are used, reporting mechanisms for IV therapy can be included for variance reporting and audit. Some suggestions are made in Table 4.3.

Table 4.3 Documenting IV therapy

Information to be recorded	Where to record it	Comments
Siting of devices		
• Type and size of device used	In electronic record, on IV therapy chart, on TPR chart	Patients' IV devices can be changed in a timely manner
• Anatomical site of device insertion	As above	Audit of practice may be undertaken at local or organisational or national level to support or develop practice on the basis of the results
• Date and time of insertion	As above	
• Name and signature of practitioner inserting the device	Patient notes with date and time	
Disposable equipment		
• Date and time tubing, administration sets, other equipment changed	Labelling on the tubing and/or record on an IV therapy chart	To facilitate the timely changing of equipment as indicated
• Name and signature of practitioner responsible	Patient notes or electronic record with date and time	

Administration of IV therapy
- Signature of practitioner administering drug
- Time drug administration commenced/ended
- Volume infused if required
- Progress of infusion/function of pump

- Effect of the therapy on the patient

Incident reporting
- Adverse effects of the therapy on the patient

Patient's prescription record

As above and on drug infusion or fluid balance chart
Fluid balance chart
Drug infusion chart or fluid balance chart, PCA record chart or blood glucose chart
As above

Patient's notes or electronic record, appropriate chart (see above) and MHRA yellow card if indicated, local incident reporting mechanisms

As a record that the prescription has been given
For reference to check if infusion running at prescribed rate
For monitoring fluid balance
To check pump function is accurate and correctly set

To ensure efficacy of the therapy, adjust therapy as indicated and prescribed or intervene if effects are adverse

To gain information about drug effects and reactions for future use with this patient and others

Table 4.3 Documenting IV therapy

Information to be recorded	Where to record it	Comments
• Infiltration or extravasation of infusion and action taken	Patient's notes and IV therapy chart, local incident reporting mechanisms	For auditing of IV therapy practice
• Phlebitis or other inflammatory or infection-related complications	As above	As above
• Accidental removal of the device	Patient's notes or electronic record with details of incident, local incident reporting mechanisms	For auditing of IV therapy practice
• Damage to a central catheter and action taken	Patient's notes or electronic record and IV therapy chart with details	To avoid recurrence
• Pump function error or damage	Local incident reporting mechanisms	

Key points

- Before administering IV therapy, understand the pathophysiology of anaphylaxis, know how to recognise it and provide first-line treatment

- Check the five 'rights' are correct before giving the drug: right patient, right drug, right dose, right time, right route

- Prepare drugs in a clean, quiet environment

- Use handwashing and asepsis at all times

- Avoid introducing drug spray into the environment

- Use the appropriate equipment and techniques to avoid contamination by micro-organisms or particles

- Ensure compatibility of drugs and infusion fluids with each other

- Use luer-lock connecting equipment to avoid disconnection and embolus

- Do not give more than one drug at a time through one VAD unless *certain* of their compatibility

- Prepare the patient for receiving the drug and its effects

- Give the drug at the appropriate speed, check infusions regularly

- Never use sedative or opiate infusions with any other infusion through the same VAD

- Use pumps when indicated, not as a short cut

- Get training on pumps and know the pumps available for patients' infusions

- Use the most appropriate pump for the patient's needs

- Check the settings when starting the infusion, when taking over the patient's care and regularly thereafter

- Monitor pumps' functioning: they cannot communicate every fault

- Clean and zero pumps' settings after use

- Keep mains/battery pumps plugged into the mains when being moved or not in use to charge the battery

- Take faulty pumps out of use and report the fault

- Document all aspects of IV therapy in patients' notes or electronic records and on the appropriate charts and equipment for continuity of care, safety and audit purposes

REFERENCES

BNF (2003) *British National Formulary*. British Medical Association & Royal Pharmaceutical Society of Great Britain, London.

Clayton, M. (1987) The right way to prevent medicine errors. *Registered Nurse*, June, 30–31.

Dolan, S. (1999) Intravenous flow control and infusion devices. In: L. Dougherty & J. Lamb eds, *Intravenous Therapy in Nursing Practice*. Churchill Livingstone, Edinburgh.

Dougherty, L. (2000a) Drug administration. In: J. Mallett & L. Dougherty, *Royal Marsden Manual of Clinical Nursing Procedures* 5th edn. Blackwell Science, Oxford.

Dougherty, L. (2000b) Infusion devices. In: J. Mallett & L. Dougherty, *Royal Marsden Manual of Clinical Nursing Procedures* 5th edn. Blackwell Science, Oxford.

Dougherty, L. (2002) Delivery of intravenous therapy. *Nursing Standard* **16**(16), 45–52.

Dougherty, L. & Lamb, J. eds (1999) *Intravenous Therapy in Nursing Practice*. Churchill Livingstone, Edinburgh.

Glenister, H. (2001) Safety tips. *Nursing Times* **97**(41), 24–25.

Nichol, M. (1999) Safe administration and management of peripheral intravenous therapy. In: L. Dougherty & J. Lamb eds, *Intravenous Therapy in Nursing Practice*. Churchill Livingstone, Edinburgh.

NMC (2002) *Guidelines for Records and Record Keeping*. Nursing and Midwifery Council, London.

Nowack, T.J. & Handford, A.G. (1999) *Essentials of Pathophysiology* 2nd edn. McGraw-Hill, Boston.

Sani, M.H. (1999) Pharmacological aspects of intravenous drug therapy. In: L. Dougherty & J. Lamb eds, *Intravenous Therapy in Nursing Practice*. Churchill Livingstone, Edinburgh.

Tait, J. (2000) Nursing management. In: H. Hamilton ed., *Total Parenteral Nutrition: a Practical Guide for Nurses*. Churchill Livingstone, Edinburgh.

Weinstein, S.M. (2001) *Plumer's Principles and Practice of Intravenous Therapy* 7th edn. Lippincott, Philadelphia.
Whyte, A. (2001) Well-equipped? *Nursing Times* **97**(42), 22–23.

ADDITIONAL TEXTS
Otto, S. (2001) *Oncology Nursing* 4th edn. Mosby, London.
Royal College of Nursing (1999) *Guidelines on the Administration of Cytotoxic Chemotherapy*. RCN, London.

WEBSITES
British National Formulary
http://www.bnf.org/index.htm

Chemotherapy administration
http://www.doh.gov.uk/cancer

Health Technology Board Scotland – reports and bulletins relating to medical equipment in Scotland
http://www.htbs.org.uk

Medicines and Healthcare products Regulatory Agency – reports and bulletins relating to medical equipment, including infusion pumps, in England
http://www.mhra.gov.uk

Nursing and Midwifery Council
http://www.nmk-uk.org

Intravenous Fluid Therapy

5

INTRODUCTION

Fluids are infused intravenously to restore or maintain fluid and electrolyte balance when it is not possible for a patient to do so independently. If a patient has experienced dehydration or injury, fluids or blood may be required intravenously to rapidly replace lost volume and regain homeostasis. For patients with haematological disorders or simple anaemia, infusing blood or blood products intravenously is crucial to their survival. The fluid administered is dependent on the needs of the patient, and an understanding of how deficits occur is important in understanding IV fluid regimens. This chapter will cover:

❏ fluid imbalances; hypervolaemia and hypovolaemia;
❏ intravenous fluid therapies; crystalloid and colloid;
❏ blood and blood products; immunology, screening and transfusion;
❏ parenteral nutrition; indications, components and administration.

FLUID IMBALANCES

Imbalance in fluid volume is due to excess or insufficient fluid volume in one or more of the fluid compartments, and is usually associated with electrolyte or acid–base imbalance, depending on the cause of the problem. Treatment is aimed at correcting the cause of the problem and assisting the body to restore fluid, electrolyte and acid–base balance with the appropriate intervention.

Hypervolaemia

This is due to fluid overload, when there is an increase in the extracellular fluid volume. In severe cases, in young children or elderly people and in patients with cardiac or renal problems, this can result in pulmonary oedema and cardiac failure. This occurs when:

(1) Sodium and water are retained due to renal, cardiac, hepatic or endocrine problems. Because the excess fluid is isotonic there is no excess *water* for the kidneys to excrete.

(2) Hypertonic intravenous fluid is infused. Infusion of hypertonic fluid draws fluid from the interstitial spaces to the circulation, thereby increasing the circulatory volume.

(3) Water alone increases the circulatory volume. This can happen if a patient is over-hydrated with 5% dextrose. The solution is initially isotonic, but the dextrose is rapidly metabolised and the remaining water in the circulation is drawn into the interstitial fluid and the cells in an effort to achieve a balance. Plasma levels of sodium and blood cells are reduced by the diluting effect of the water (see Table 5.1).

Signs and symptoms

- Weight gain and peripheral oedema (sacral oedema in bed- or chair-bound patients).
- Bounding pulse due to high cardiac output.
- Proportionally higher fluid intake than output, i.e. a positive fluid balance greater than 500 ml per 24 hours.
- Raised jugular venous pressure.
- Raised central venous pressure.
- Dyspnoea and cyanosis due to pulmonary oedema.

Treatment is primarily aimed at relieving the circulatory overload. This is achieved by restricting fluid (water and sodium) intake and/or the administration of diuretics to inhibit the reabsorption of sodium and water by the kidney. Careful monitoring of the patient's electrolyte levels, weight, fluid balance and cardio-respiratory function (BP, heart rate, CVP, respiratory rate and oxygen saturation) is important to avoid inadequate or excessive diuresis and electrolyte loss. Hypokalaemia and hyponatraemia are side effects of diuretic therapy (see Table 2.2) with potentially dangerous implications. Supplements of potassium may be necessary for patients on high-dose or long-term diuretic therapy. Patients in renal failure may need dialysis.

Intravenous fluid infusions must be carefully managed in order to prevent the possibility of fluid overload occurring.

Hypovolaemia

This is the loss of water and/or electrolytes and blood proteins from one or more compartments. It can occur for a number of reasons and people at extremes of age are much more susceptible to smaller changes.

(1) Diarrhoea and vomiting, or haemorrhage will result in the loss of fluids and electrolytes from the circulating volume.

(2) Simple dehydration arises when water intake is reduced, as in those unable to ask for a drink, or in the elderly whose thirst reflex is impaired. Patients with diabetes insipidus will lose large volumes of water in dilute urine due to a lack of antidiuretic hormone production from the pituitary gland. When water from insensible losses, including respiration, is not replaced, dehydration occurs.

(3) The loss of fluid rich in electrolytes causes hypovolaemia. These include
- Increased urine output induced by diuretics.
- Losses from the gut via bowel fistulae, ileostomies, vomiting or nasogastric tube drainage or diarrhoea.

- Excessive sweating or diaphoresis.
- Third spacing of body fluids. This is the collection of fluids in a part of the body where they are not usually held, and from which they are not readily absorbed. Their movement and 'loss' from their usual compartments is hidden and symptoms of hypovolaemia can arise without immediately obvious excretion of fluid. Third spacing occurs with paralytic ileus (electrolyte-rich fluid is secreted into the gut but not reabsorbed – see Table 2.3), ascites and peritonitis and following surgery.

Signs and symptoms

- Weight loss.
- Weakness and lethargy.
- Negative fluid balance; often, but not always with reduced urine output.
- Increased heart rate and weak, thready pulse.
- Reduced blood pressure.

All types of hypovolaemia require replacement, often intravenously, and the regimen chosen will depend on the cause of the problem and the type of fluid lost. Treatment will aim to replace the fluid lost in quantity and quality and, where necessary, substitute for normal intake. Where haemorrhage has occurred, plasma-expanding colloids and blood will be transfused to increase the circulatory volume and oxygen transport (see Table 5.2). Patients with simple dehydration may be treated with 5% dextrose infusion, whilst those undergoing gastrointestinal surgery may be prescribed a regimen of dextrose saline with additional potassium to replace lost water and electrolytes. (See Table 5.1 for commonly used crystalloid solutions and their uses.)

INTRAVENOUS FLUID THERAPIES

Fluids are administered intravenously to patients, taking into account their previous state of fluid and electrolyte balance

Table 5.1 Common crystalloids and their characteristics (Malster 1999, Weinstein 2001)

Solution	Content in water	Tonicity	Fluid space	Indications
Normal saline 0.9% sodium chloride solution	Na$^+$ 150 mmol/l Cl$^-$ 150 mmol/l	Isotonic	Circulating blood volume and interstitial fluid	Rehydration, increasing extracellular fluid volume
Dextrose saline Dextrose 4% Sodium chloride 0.18%	Glucose 40 g Na$^+$ 30 mmol/l Cl$^-$ 30 mmol/l	Isotonic	All fluid compartments	Fluid balance maintenance
5% dextrose	Glucose 50 g	Isotonic	All fluid compartments	Water replacement Patients requiring low sodium intake e.g. liver failure
Compound sodium lactate (Ringer's lactate or Hartmann's solution)	Na$^+$ 131 mmol/l Cl$^-$ 111 mmol/l Ca$^+$ 2.0 mmol/l K$^+$ 5 mmol/l Lactate 29 mmol/l	Isotonic	Circulating blood volume and interstitial fluid	A solution of water and electrolytes mimicking body fluid including bicarbonate ions (metabolised lactate). Used in hydration and perioperatively.

and their existing needs for maintenance and replacement therapy.

Crystalloid

These fluids are solutions of electrolytes in water and vary in their content. They may be hypotonic, isotonic or hypertonic to blood plasma. Depending on their content they will expand the extracellular fluid volume or the intracellular fluid volume, or both (see Table 5.1). Isotonic solutions may be infused rapidly (whilst monitoring the patient's response); hypertonic (10% glucose, parenteral nutrition) and hypotonic solutions (0.45% sodium chloride) must be infused slowly and carefully to avoid water shift into the extracellular fluid and haemolysis, respectively. Hypertonic solutions are likely to be irritant to the veins and cause thrombophlebitis, thus are preferably infused into large central veins to facilitate mixing and dilution with the circulating blood (Weinstein 2001).

Crystalloid may be given through standard administration sets, depending on the rate of infusion required. Blood administration sets have a wider bore and facilitate more rapid infusion in emergency situations.

Colloid

Colloid solutions all contain large molecules dissolved in water. All colloid solutions are hypertonic and are used to expand the circulatory blood volume and raise blood pressure in shock from burns, septicaemia or hypovolaemia. They stay in the circulation and, being hypertonic, exert osmotic pressure on the interstitial fluid, drawing it into the circulation (see Table 5.2). Patients being given colloid solutions need to be *monitored carefully for fluid overload*. Colloid solutions have no oxygen-carrying capacity. The preferred administration set is usually a blood administration set to allow rapid infusion when necessary. In addition, the 170 micron filter in the set is necessary for filtering out particles in the blood products.

Table 5.2 Common colloids and their characteristics (Malster 1999, Porter 1999, Weinstein 2001)

Solution	Content	Notes
Dextrans	Polysaccharides of low or high molecular weight (LMW or HMW) in solution with 0.9% sodium chloride or 5% dextrose	Dextran 40 (LMW) is used for patients with peripheral vascular problems, not for volume replacement Dextran 70 or 110 (HMW) (in 0.9% sodium chloride) is used for hypotension or hypovolaemia, for burns or shocked patients Anaphylactoid reactions occur more often, patients need close monitoring Excreted renally
Hetastarch (Hespan)	6% solution of starch molecules in 0.9% sodium chloride	Interferes with coagulation Less risk of anaphylaxis Excreted renally, contraindicated in renal failure
Gelatine (Gelofusine, Haemaccel)	4% solution of gelatine molecules in approximately 0.9% sodium chloride	Excreted renally
Human albumin solution (HAS)	Isotonic = 5% solution of human proteins derived from plasma (heat treated) Hypertonic = 20% solution	Replacement of lost plasma volume (burns, pancreatitis, trauma, post-operatively) Hypoalbuminaemia Hypoalbuminaemia in liver failure, used in conjunction with sodium and water restriction to reduce oedema
Plasma protein fraction (PPF)	Human plasma protein solution (heat treated)	Increase the circulating volume
Fresh frozen plasma (FFP)	Plasma containing clotting factors, separated from whole blood and frozen	Must be ABO and Rh compatible To correct clotting deficiencies (liver disease, DIC, following massive transfusion)

BLOOD AND BLOOD PRODUCTS

Whole blood or any of its constituents may be transfused into a patient who is deficient in the constituent being given. Transfusion therapy has become much more common and safe in recent decades and many modern treatments are reliant on the use of transfusions for their existence. These include cardiac and transplant surgery, bone marrow transplant, and high-dose chemotherapy regimens. Whole blood is made up of a number of constituents (see Fig. 5.1), the properties and actions of which must be understood in order to safely administer blood and blood product transfusion.

Immunology and compatibility

Like most cells in the body, blood cell membranes contain proteins that act as antigenic markers. These antigens identify the cells to the immune system as 'self' or foreign, foreign ones inducing immune 'rejection-type' chemical responses. There are many different groups of antigens carried on blood cell surfaces; the two principal markers are the ABO antigens and the Rhesus antigen, both carried on the red blood cells. White blood cells' principal antigen is the human leucocytic antigen (HLA). In blood transfusion, donor blood is matched to

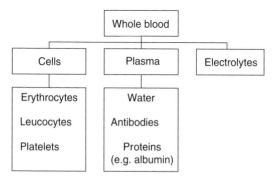

Fig. 5.1 Constituents of whole blood

recipients' ABO and RhesusD antigens, or blood group, as well as to other significant antibodies.

ABO types

Blood types, the antigens expressed on the cell membranes, are inherited genetically. The ABO antigens mean that an individual has either A or B antigens or both, or neither. Individuals with the O blood group have neither A nor B antigens. Those born with A or B antigens make antibodies to the other antigen during infancy. This means that if red blood cells with the other antigen enter their body (by a mismatched transfusion, for example) their antibodies will attack the 'foreign' red blood cells though they ignore the person's own red blood cells. For example, a person who has the blood group A will express A antigen on their red blood cells. They will have made anti-B antibodies as a baby. If they are then given blood (or tissue in a transplant) from a Type B or a Type AB person, their antibodies will attack the B or AB marked cells because they are recognised as foreign. A person who is Type AB will not have any antibodies to the ABO type at all. A person who is Type O will have anti-A and anti-B antibodies. The antibodies attack by binding to the foreign cells' antigen. The antigen/antibody complex attracts components of a chemical called complement, which also bind to the cell resulting in its lysis and death. This occurs in the bloodstream and can have serious, potentially fatal, consequences for the patient (see Table 5.3).

RhesusD types

Similarly to the ABO system, everyone has a RhesusD type that is governed by the presence or absence of the RhesusD antigen on their red blood cells. Those with the D antigen are called RhesusD positive; those without are RhesusD negative. Compatibility of RhesusD types is also vital, though a reaction to an incompatible type happens in a different way from the

Table 5.3 ABO blood types compatibility

Blood type	Antigens on red blood cells	Antibodies in recipient's body	Compatible types	Incompatible types
A	A	Anti B	A, O	B
B	B	Anti A	B, O	A
AB	AB	None	A, B, AB, O	None
O	None	Anti-A & anti-B	O	A, B, AB

ABO types. A person who is RhesusD positive has no antibodies to the D antigen and they can receive blood with or without the D antigen, that is, RhesusD positive or negative blood. A person who is RhesusD negative has no D antigens, but nor do they make anti-D antibodies automatically. However, if they are given RhesusD positive blood, or are exposed to it in some way such as in childbirth, the B cells in their immune system will make anti-D antibodies for future use. Should the person receive or be exposed to RhesusD positive blood again, the anti-D antibodies will attack the RhesusD positive blood cells in the same way described earlier for the ABO types. (See Table 5.4 for Rhesus compatibility.) For this reason, donors' blood types are identified and their donated blood clearly marked with the type at the time of the donation.

It is always preferable to give crossmatched, compatible blood to a patient to minimise the occurrence of any transfusion reaction, however minor. In emergency situations it is possible to give a patient blood that is not crossmatched. In extreme emergencies, any patient can be given Type O, Rhesus negative blood. Where blood is needed within 15 minutes the patient may be given blood that is of the same type as theirs (it can be tested for the type in that time) without the donor

Table 5.4 Rhesus blood types compatibility

Blood type	Antigens on red blood cells	Anti-D antibodies	Compatible types
RhesusD positive (RhD +ve)	D antigens	None	RhD +ve and RhD −ve
RhesusD negative (RhD −ve)	None	Only after first exposure to RhD +ve blood	RhD −ve only

blood being fully crossmatched. Fully crossmatched blood requires an hour or more for testing (Contreras & Mollison 1998).

Screening

In the United Kingdom, blood donors, all of whom are very carefully screened for high-risk behaviours associated with blood-borne infections, donate blood free. Before donating blood, donors are asked about high-risk activities, including active male homosexuality, intravenous drug use, international travel and body piercing or accidental needle-stick injury. Involvement in any of these activities or incidents will mean exclusion from donating blood, on either a permanent or a temporary basis depending on the activity concerned, because of the significantly increased risk of transmission of disease through the blood.

In addition, donors' blood is screened for HIV, hepatitis B antigen, hepatitis C and *Treponema pallidum* (syphilis). Cytomegalovirus (CMV) and specific antibodies are screened for in blood to be given to inmmunocompromised patients in order to reduce the risk of blood-borne disease transmission between donors and recipients. More specific screening of donor blood can be carried out if needed for a recipient with particular needs (Hewitt & Wagstaff 1998).

Transfusion

People who are to receive blood will be tested for their blood type and also screened for antibodies as donors are. Not all blood products are matched between donor and recipient; potential reaction to blood products depends on the principal antigen/antibody matching on red blood cells. Not all blood products without red blood cells need to be matched for donor–recipient compatibility (see Table 5.5). Before having a transfusion of blood or blood products, patients should, where at all possible, be consulted and informed about the need for the transfusion, the associated risks and benefits, and be supported in giving informed consent to the transfusion.

Checking the transfusion for a patient is crucial to avoid the wrong blood or blood product being given to a patient and causing a potentially life-threatening reaction. Two people should check the blood product and the patient's details; one of these must be a registered nurse or a doctor. When a patient is prescribed a transfusion of a blood product the infusion must be collected from the storage fridge and used within the time specified, which will depend on the product in question (see Table 5.5). The checking procedure should cover the following:

- the patient's identity and that on the prescription and the crossmatch report must all be identical;
- the blood product must be correctly prescribed;
- for transfusions where crossmatching is required, the patient's blood group (on the crossmatch report) and that of the pack of blood to be transfused, must be the same, or at least compatible for transfusions given in an emergency;
- the donation number on the crossmatch report and that on the pack of blood must be identical;

Table 5.5 Blood products: uses and administration guidance (Porter 1999)

Blood product	Constituents	Rationale for prescription	Volume per pack (approx.)	Compatibility required	Administration sets	Administration techniques
Whole blood	All those of blood.	Transfusion to replace lost cells and volume.	450 ml	Crossmatch	Blood administration set. Change sets after two units.	Commence transfusion within 30 minutes of removal from fridge. Never return to fridge. Give at prescribed rate, not longer than five hours.
Packed cells	Plasma-reduced, concentration of cells.	Transfusion to replace lost red cells in anaemia without replacing volume.	270 ml	Crossmatch	Blood-giving set. Change sets after two units.	Commence transfusion within 30 minutes of removal from fridge. Never return to fridge. Give at prescribed rate, not longer than five hours
Platelets	Platelet concentrate from one or more blood donors.	Platelet dysfunction. Thrombocytopaenia due to: (1) Bone marrow failure. (2) Dilution with massive transfusion.	50–70 ml	ABO and Rhesus compatibility preferable	Platelet infusion set or inject as a bolus. Blood-giving sets and microfilters can damage the platelets.	Infuse as fast as possible. Use within three days of donation.

Product	Description	Indications	Volume	Compatibility	Administration set	Notes
Fresh frozen plasma	Blood plasma including clotting factors and additional fibrinogen, frozen within eight hours of collection.	Coagulation disorders, inherited or acquired. Following massive blood transfusions.	180–200 ml	ABO and Rhesus compatibility	Blood-giving set, changed 12 hourly or when transfusion complete.	Transfuse as soon as possible after thawing, preferably within six hours. Give at prescribed rate.
Granulocytes	Granulocytes separated from whole blood.	Seldom used. Persistent sepsis in neutropaenic patients.	Variable	ABO and HLA compatibility	Blood-giving set, changed 12 hourly or when transfusion complete.	Transfuse within 6–24 hours of donation at prescribed rate. Reactions are more likely and tend to be more severe.
Cryoprecipitate	Concentrate from thawed plasma containing factor VIII, von Willebrand factor and fibrinogen.	Occasionally given for specific clotting disorders or following massive blood transfusion.	Variable	ABO compatibility	Blood-giving set or platelet-giving set, changed 12 hourly or when transfusion complete.	Transfuse within six hours of thawing.
Human albumin solution	5% solution of human albumin.	Replacement of lost plasma volume in burns,	500 ml	None	Standard administration set, filter not	As prescribed. Use air inlet set to vent glass bottles, Apply bottle-hanger before

Table 5.5 *Continued*

Blood product	Constituents	Rationale for prescription	Volume per pack (approx.)	Compatibility required	Administration sets	Administration techniques
		pancreatitis, trauma or postoperatively, hypoalbuminaemia.			required. Blood-giving set for rapid infusion.	connecting giving set, be vigilant to avoid air embolus at the end of the infusion. Often given in conjunction with diuretics to excrete the fluid pulled into the circulation by the osmotic pressure exerted by the albumin.
	20% solution of human albumin with reduced sodium and chloride. Both are heat-treated.	Hypoalbuminaemia in liver failure with ascites, used in conjunction with sodium and water restriction. Nephrotic syndrome with oedema.	100 ml			
Plasma protein fraction (PPF)	Less pure solution of plasma proteins than albumin. Heat-treated.	Increase blood volume.	Variable	None	As above	As prescribed.

- the expiry date on the pack of blood must not have passed;
- the pack must be checked for any signs of leaking, and not used if a leak is found (Porter 1999).

Blood may be given through a central venous catheter. Where there is more than one lumen available for the transfusion, it is recommended that the lumen with a larger diameter be used to facilitate flow of viscous blood through the catheter and prevent damage to the blood cells.

Blood must always be given alone, through dedicated venous access, and no drugs must ever be given with a blood transfusion. Blood should never be warmed up, other than by using a specially designed blood warmer.

Monitoring the patient's clinical condition during a transfusion is important in order to detect signs of a reaction as early as possible. Patient monitoring should commence before the infusion and continue until it is completed. The patient's temperature and pulse should be measured and recorded. This is repeated every 15 minutes for the first half an hour of each pack of the infusion, and hourly thereafter until the whole transfusion is complete. The packs and infusion set(s) should be kept until the whole transfusion is complete so that in the event of the patient experiencing a reaction, they may be sent to the haematology department for analysis and diagnosis of the cause of the reaction.

Crossmatched blood may still result in reactions to the transfused blood. This is due to the presence of 'foreign' antigen of types additional to those already described, contamination of the blood by micro-organisms, or fluid and electrolyte imbalance from the volume of transfusion or components of the donated blood (Porter 1999). Reactions to transfusions may result in any of the following symptoms, due to an immune system response, or lysis of the foreign cells. In massive transfusions, fluid or electrolyte imbalance and infusion of micro-aggregates (blood cells and fibrin) cause severe symptoms:

- fever;
- hypothermia;
- rigors;
- headache;
- nausea and vomiting;
- diarrhoea;
- urticaria (rash) and/or itching;
- flushing;
- pain at the site of infusion;
- back ache in the lumbar region;
- haemoglobinuria;
- disseminated intravascular coagulation (DIC);
- pulmonary oedema;
- adult respiratory distress syndrome (ARDS);
- collapse and cardiac arrest.

Despite the small risk now associated with cross-infection by blood product transfusion, some patients will refuse blood transfusions or at least be very anxious about receiving them. It is important to help them understand the implications of transfusion or refusal of transfusion, whilst providing support and appreciation for their point of view. Patients may choose to be transfused with their own blood if the circumstances allow. This may be achieved by a patient 'donating' blood up to five weeks before they undergo the procedure requiring a transfusion. Whilst this would avoid cross-infection, the risk of septicaemia from the stored blood is not insignificant. Alternatively, blood can be salvaged during surgery, washed, mixed with an anticoagulant and then re-infused. This may cause delayed haemorrhage after surgery, due to the anti-coagulants used, and is contraindicated for patients with sepsis or malignancy (Weinstein 2001).

PARENTERAL NUTRITION

Intravenous infusion of parenteral nutrition solution cannot be equated with routine intravenous fluid infusion. Patients receiving parenteral nutrition (PN), or intravenous feeding, require management by a specialist team in conjunction with the nursing and medical teams responsible for their ongoing care. This section of the chapter aims to give readers a background understanding of what parenteral nutrition is from the perspective of intravenous therapy. It is envisaged that further study, education and practice experience with a competent colleague and specialist practitioner are required to achieve competent practice in managing patients receiving PN.

Indications for parenteral nutrition therapy

In a healthy adult, normal metabolism is achieved with a balance between anabolic and catabolic reactions in the body:

- *anabolic* chemical reactions are those which use energy to convert simple substances into complex ones;
- *catabolic* chemical reactions break down complex substances to release energy.

In severe illness or lack of available nutrients, *hypercatabolism* results; muscle and fat are broken down in the face of inadequate energy availability from nutrition.

There is a fine balance to be achieved between preventing or correcting malnutrition or nutritional deficits, and not resorting to parenteral nutrition unnecessarily. Essentially, the gut is the best way to achieve nutritional balance: 'when the gut works, use it' (Weinstein 2001, p 354) is sound advice. Parenteral nutrition is potentially very risky for patients receiving it, is markedly more time consuming for all the staff involved in the patients' management and is considerably more expensive than enteral or oral nutrition.

The decision to give parenteral nutrition to a patient is based on the ability of their gut to absorb adequate nutrients for their current metabolic state, either temporarily or permanently. If they are, or will be, unable to absorb sufficient nutrients from the gut for five to seven days or more, parenteral nutrition therapy may be considered. Some patients will require feeding parenterally for only a short time of days to weeks, whilst others may be dependent on parenteral nutrition for the rest of their lives. There are many reasons for giving patients parenteral nutrition therapy and they include:

- burns, sepsis or trauma, when patients may have an excessive need for protein and calories which cannot be met by oral or enteral intake alone;
- acute pancreatitis, when patients' need for protein and calories is high and oral or enteral intake is contraindicated;
- prolonged paralytic ileus, when the bowel is not absorbing;
- inflammatory bowel disease, when oral or enteral intake is contraindicated and nutritional needs are high due to the inflammatory process, and there may be a reduced length of functional small bowel;
- enteral fistulae, when oral or enteral intake is contraindicated in order that the fistulae may heal;
- short bowel syndrome, when the patient has insufficient length of small bowel to absorb sufficient nutrients;
- cancer chemotherapy or radiotherapy, when the patient is unable to take oral or enteral feeding due to severe mucositis or radiation enteritis;
- intractable vomiting and diarrhoea, when oral or enteral intake is impossible and nutritional, fluid and electrolyte needs are high;
- hyperemesis gravidarum (severe vomiting in pregnancy), when oral or enteral intake is impossible;
- AIDs, when the patient is unable to take oral or enteral feeding and nutritional needs are high (Burnham 1999, Pennington 2000, Weinstein 2001).

Components of PN

Parenteral nutrition aims to supply those aspects of a patient's nutrition which they cannot achieve independently. For many this includes the whole spectrum of nutrients, including:

- glucose;
- lipids;
- amino acids;
- vitamins;
- electrolytes;
- trace elements;
- water.

Energy requirements are met using glucose and fats. Glucose is the source of energy in carbohydrate form. The drawbacks of using glucose for energy needs are:

- high levels of glucose require large volumes of water for dilution and cause thrombophlebitis due to its hypertonic nature;
- hyperglycaemia;
- increased CO_2 levels from glucose metabolism, which can cause dyspnoea or problems weaning from a ventilator, and acid–base imbalance.

Lipid solutions contain essential fatty acids and can provide a high energy nutrient source in less volume. They are used to supply up to 50% of energy needs in parenteral nutrition solutions. Their inclusion moderates the hypertonic effect of high glucose concentrations.

Amino acids are supplied in synthetic crystalline form to achieve the required nitrogen balance. Vitamins are usually added to the solution just before it is administered, in compound solutions. There are two main groups of vitamins, those which are water soluble and those which are fat soluble. Some vitamins degrade quickly due to temperature change, light exposure (Vitamin A) or oxidation (Vitamin C) and the use of covers and layered bags can reduce this (Pennington 2000). Trace elements or micronutrients have been shown to be important, particularly for severely malnourished patients, and are included in a trace element solution. They include:

- iron;
- zinc;
- manganese;
- selenium;
- copper;
- chromium;
- iodine;
- fluorine;
- cobalt;
- molybdenum.

Electrolytes are usually included in standard quantities, although these may be varied according to individual patients' specific needs. More may be added for patients who have fluid and electrolyte-rich losses from fistulae or ileostomies. Other patients will require electrolyte levels to be reduced, if there is sodium retention or renal failure, for example.

Preparation of parenteral nutrition solutions

Parenteral nutrition solutions are prepared specially by pharmacists in sterile, laminar-flow cabinets to avoid contamination; clearly the constituents of parenteral nutrition provide ideal nutrients to micro-organisms as well as to the people they are intended for. The prescribed content of the individual patient's infusion is reconstituted particularly so that the solution is stable. The infusion should not be added to after it has left the pharmacy, as this may affect the compatibility of the components and the stability of the solution. (There are circumstances where this is unavoidable if drugs can only be added immediately before administration and bags are already prepared. Drugs should only be added by an expert practitioner using strict aseptic technique.)

The solution must be stored in a refrigerator at 1–4°C until it is to be infused, preferably in a refrigerator dedicated to PN storage to avoid contamination.

IV access for parenteral nutrition

Parenteral nutrition is usually given into a central venous catheter, particularly if it is required for longer than two weeks. It is possible to administer parenteral nutrition through a peripheral cannula. It is less risky for the patient but it is important that the parenteral nutrition solution contains lipid and preferably less glucose so as to reduce the thrombophlebitis associated with administering hypertonic glucose solutions into peripheral veins. The cannula site must be monitored very carefully and re-sited regularly in a large vein every 48 hours, and immediately if phlebitis has occurred.

Dedicated, single-lumen central venous catheters and peripherally inserted central catheters are more commonly used to administer parenteral nutrition to patients. If the therapy is expected to continue for a prolonged period, a tunnelled, cuffed central venous catheter will need to be inserted (Hamilton 2000a). This procedure is risky for the patient both during and after the insertion of the catheter. It is imperative that the tip of the catheter is checked for position in the central venous system prior to commencing any infusion. Information on the potential risks and recommended care of patients' CVCs is detailed in Chapter 3.

Patients who are to have parenteral nutrition therapy should have this aspect of their care managed by a specialist team in conjunction with the health care professionals caring for them in their existing illness. This team includes:

- specialist nurse;
- dietician;
- pharmacist;
- specialist doctor (Hudson 2000).

The patient should have the implications of line insertion, feeding with parenteral nutrition and why they require it, clearly explained to them in advance so that they may give an informed consent to the procedures involved. It may be helpful for some patients who are likely to have the therapy for several weeks or longer, to meet a patient who has experience of parenteral nutrition therapy and to discuss the implications of it with them.

Administering parenteral nutrition

It is important that practitioners involved in caring for patients with parenteral nutrition and managing their infusions have the additional skills and knowledge to do this. Running parenteral nutrition therapy is not the same as giving a patient any other intravenous fluid infusion. The potential risks are significant and care must incorporate suitable assessment and monitoring to facilitate early detection and prevention of serious complications, with clear communication between all the professionals involved in the patients' care. In addition to the complications associated with infection, phlebitis and catheter damage or occlusion, patients having parenteral nutrition are at risk of metabolic complications associated with the infusion (see Table 5.6). These are often avoidable when regimens are carefully prescribed and administered with close monitoring of the patient.

Every effort must be made to maintain the sterility of the solution and administration sets, and parenteral nutrition must be given through a *dedicated vascular access device* (a catheter used only for the parenteral nutrition infusion) to minimise the risk of contamination or destabilising the solution. The catheter should not be manipulated other than when changing the infusion, which must be undertaken using strict aseptic technique. A volumetric pump must be used to run the infusion, as a consistent rate of administration is vital to avoid metabolic complications associated with excessive or intermittent flow rates, principally inconsistent glucose levels. The

Table 5.6 Potential complications of PN administration; causes and indications for patient monitoring (Burnham 1999, Hamilton 2000b, Weinstein 2001)

Complications	Monitoring (to avoid or detect early)
Infection Increased incidence due to: (1) Presence of catheter into central venous system. (2) Constituents of infusion. (3) Patient's depressed T cell production. (4) High level of free radical production with PN metabolism. (5) Micronutrient deficiency with PN. • Catheter-related septicaemia. • Skin/catheter exit site infection. • Catheter tunnel infection.	• *Strict use of aseptic technique at all times* when handling the catheter, site, or infusion. • Temperature, pulse and respiratory rate (TPR) six hourly. • TPR twice daily when stable. • Immediately if signs and symptoms develop.
Mechanical • Thrombosis, potentially life-threatening complication leading to pulmonary embolism. Exacerbated by high glucose solution and lipid emulsions, and large catheters in small veins.	• TPR as above. • Blood pressure monitoring if the patient is unstable or signs and symptoms indicate. • Respiratory rate and oxygen saturation if the patient develops respiratory distress or chest pain.

Table 5.6 *Continued*

Complications	Monitoring (to avoid or detect early)
	• Catheter occlusion pinching, fibrin, lipid sludge or other debris.	• Monitoring infusion rates and patency of the catheter when flushing.
• Fracturing of the catheter or hub/port.	• Minimise handling of catheter and by experienced personnel only. Clamps and scissors should not be used on, or in the vicinity of, central venous catheters. Can be mended.
• Disconnection between port and catheter.	• Patients with implanted ports may complain of pain at the port site. Stop infusion and refer for expert intervention.
	• Can be replaced or mended depending or catheter type.
Metabolic	• Hyperglycamia This may be more likely in 'stressed' patients or those who have been malnourished prior	• Check blood sugar 12 hourly, daily serum blood sugar until stable.
	• When stable check urine daily, twice weekly serum blood glucose test.

- Check blood sugar if symptoms indicate a change (thirst, oliguria, weakness, sweating, nausea, confusion, altered consciousness).
- Increase frequency of blood sugar monitoring if insulin infusion is required.
- As above.

- Blood test after 24 hours of PN infusion.
- Weigh daily (at the same time, in the same clothes, on the same scales).
- Keep accurate fluid balance charts recording all intake and output until the patient's condition is stable.
- Daily serum urea, electrolyte levels and osmolality until stable and then twice weekly.
- 24 hour urine collections twice weekly.

to PN commencing or if the rate of infusion is increased. Rate of PN infusions *should not be increased* to 'catch up'.

- Hypoglycaemia. Likely if feed is abruptly stopped. It should always be tapered and the patient more closely monitored when a cycled regimen is commenced (e.g. feeding overnight or on alternate days).

- Lipaemia.
- Fluid and electrolyte imbalance.

Table 5.6 *Continued*

Complications	Monitoring (to avoid or detect early)
• Hypomagnesaemia. Hypophosphataemia. Hypokalaemia. All result in re-feeding syndrome. Malnourished patients started on PN may experience the life-threatening effects of these electrolyte changes as their energy source changes from ketones to glucose and cellular uptake of these electrolytes occurs (serum levels drop).	• Monitoring of serum magnesium and phosphate in addition to routine electrolytes daily initially or if re-feeding suspected (confusion, thrombocytopaenia, cardiac disrhythmias and cardiac arrest).
• Insufficient trace elements.	• Serum level when PN commenced. • Serum levels every 6 to 12 weeks depending on the patient's condition and the amounts infused.
• Altered liver function due to high levels of glucose infusion.	• Liver function tests, full blood counts and coagulation screen every three to four days.

pump must have occlusion, air-in-line, and 'volume infused' alarms (see p 135), and should not allow free flow of solution (Pennington 2000).

When the patient is able, oral and/or enteral intake should be introduced and increased until a sufficient amount of food of appropriate nutritional value can be taken. A detailed record of the patient's intake must be kept so that analysis of the protein, calorie, fat and other nutritional components can be estimated. On the basis of this estimation and the patient's progress more generally, a plan to reduce and then stop the parenteral infusion can be made by the specialist team. Parenteral infusions are never abruptly stopped because of rebound hypoglycaemia (see Table 5.6). When the patient is ready to stop parenteral feeding the feed is weaned by gradually decreasing the rate of the infusion over days (Burnham 1999).

Key points

- IV fluid infusion is aimed at correcting imbalance to restore fluid, electrolyte and acid–base balance or to maintain homeostasis when the patient is unable to do so independently

- Crystalloid is a fluid solution of electrolytes in water that may be isotonic, hypertonic or hypotonic with blood, depending on its constituents

- Colloid is a solution of large molecules dissolved in water; always hypertonic, colloid expands the plasma volume and increases blood pressure

- Whole blood and its constituents can be transfused into a patient who is haemorrhaging or deficient in a specific constituent

- ABO and RhD type matching is preferable as a minimum; in emergencies, Type O Rh –ve blood may be given to anyone

- Blood and blood products must be stored, checked and administered only as directed to avoid life-threatening reactions in the patient or damage to the donated blood product

- Parenteral nutrition is not a routine fluid or food replacement; knowledge and understanding of its implications for patient care are essential

- If the gut works, use it

- Parenteral nutrition must never be added to once prepared and must be stored appropriately in a refrigerator

- Parenteral nutrition must be administered through dedicated IV access, preferably a CVAD, and handled by practitioners with the necessary skills and knowledge

- Parenteral nutrition infusion rates must not be altered without prescription; the patient may experience sudden metabolic changes due to hyperglycaemia or hypoglycaemia

- Patients should be weaned off parenteral nutrition only when they are able to absorb adequate protein and calories enterally

REFERENCES

Burnham, P. (1999). Parenteral nutrition. In: L. Dougherty & J. Lamb eds, *Intravenous Therapy in Nursing Practice.* Churchill Livingstone, Edinburgh.

Calhoun, L. (1989) Blood product preparation and administration. In: L.D. Petz & S.N. Swisher eds, *Clinical Practice of Transfusion Medicine* 2nd edn. Churchill Livingstone, New York.

Contreras, M. & Mollison, P.L. (1998) Testing before transfusion and blood ordering policies. In: M. Contreras ed., *ABC of Transfusion* 3rd edn. British Medical Journal Books, London.

Hamilton, H. (2000a) Choosing the appropriate catheter. In: H. Hamilton ed., *Total Parenteral Nutrition: a Practical Guide for Nurses.* Churchill Livingstone, Edinburgh.

Hamilton, H. ed. (2000b) *Total Parenteral Nutrition: a Practical Guide for Nurses.* Churchill Livingstone, Edinburgh.

Hewitt, P. & Wagstaff, W. (1998) The blood donor and tests on donor blood. In: M. Contreras ed., *ABC of Transfusion* 3rd edn. British Medical Journal Books, London.

Hoy, S. (2000) Blood transfusion. In: J. Mallett & L. Dougherty eds, *Royal Marsden Hospital Manual of Clinical Nursing Procedures* 5th edn. Blackwell Science, Oxford.

Hudson, J. (2000) The multidisciplinary team. In: H. Hamilton ed., *Total Parenteral Nutrition: a Practical Guide for Nurses*. Churchill Livingstone, Edinburgh.

Malster, M. (1999) Fluid and electrolyte balance. In: L. Dougherty & J. Lamb eds, *Intravenous Therapy in Nursing Practice*. Churchill Livingstone, Edinburgh.

Pennington, C. (2000) What is parenteral nutrition? In: H. Hamilton ed., *Total Parenteral Nutrition: a Practical Guide for Nurses*. Churchill Livingstone, Edinburgh.

Porter, H. (1999) Blood transfusion therapy. In: L. Dougherty & J. Lamb eds, *Intravenous Therapy in Nursing Practice*. Churchill Livingstone, Edinburgh.

Tait, J. (2000) Nursing management. In: H. Hamilton ed., *Total Parenteral Nutrition: a Practical Guide for Nurses*. Churchill Livingstone, Edinburgh.

Weinstein, S.M. (2001) *Plumer's Principles and Practice of Intravenous Therapy* 7th edn. Lippincott, Philadelphia.

WEBSITES

British Association for Parenteral and Enteral Nutrition – information and publications
http://www.bapen.org.uk

Department of Health Site on blood transfusion – includes guidelines and links
http://www.doh.gov.uk/blood/bbt.htm

Guidelines for blood transfusion
http://transfusionguidelines.org.uk

Pharmacology and Intravenous Therapy

6

INTRODUCTION

Pharmacology is the study of drugs, their chemical structure, different preparations and their administration, drug actions, metabolism and excretion. Practitioners administering intravenous therapy must have the knowledge and competence to do so, as detailed in Chapter 1. This consists of knowledge of the fundamental principles of pharmacology including pharmacodynamics – how drugs act – and pharmacokinetics – how drugs are dealt with by the body. Knowledge of potential risks, including those due to interactions and drug incompatibilities, informs practice in intravenous therapy, as does a good working knowledge of fundamental mathematics in order that drug doses and infusion volumes can be safely calculated. This chapter covers:

❏ pharmacodynamics; how drugs act in the body;
❏ pharmacokinetics; how the body deals with drugs;
❏ monitoring drug levels and effects;
❏ timings of intravenous drug administration;
❏ the implications of using the intravenous route;
❏ calculations; units, formulae, percentages and ratios;
❏ test calculations; answers at the end of the chapter;
❏ information resources for drugs and their administration.

PHARMACODYNAMICS

It is likely that almost all drugs act by interfering with cell activity in some way, or they replace deficient chemicals that are involved in cell activity. Despite significant advances in pharmacological and physiological research, the specific action of many drugs is still not clearly understood. However, most commonly administered drugs act in one of the following ways.

Replacement

Where a person is deficient in certain substances used by the body, these may be substituted; this is likely to be a life-long therapeutic need, such as in people with diabetes or under-active thyroid function. Vitamins and minerals are also supplemented when these are deficient or higher levels are required than the patient is able to take or absorb.

Receptor binding

Receptors are protein molecules on cell membranes with specific structures. In a 'lock and key' fashion, receptors and chemicals (sometimes known as ligands) combine and produce an effect as a result of their binding. For example, acetylcholine binds with receptors on muscle cells and stimulates the muscle to contract. Some drugs directly replace the receptors' naturally occurring ligand, bind with it and produce the same effect. These are known as *agonists*. Other drugs bind the receptors without producing the desired effect, and prevent them being bound by the natural ligand, blocking the receptors' usual function. These are called *antagonists*.

For example, morphine sulphate and diamorphine are agonists which bind opioid receptors to produce analgesic effects. Naloxone is an antagonist for opioid receptors, binding them to block analgesic effect.

Enzymes

Protein molecules that enhance chemical reactions in the body are known as enzymes. Some drugs act by blocking the effects of enzymes, thus reducing the level of chemical reaction and its effect.

For example, enzymes facilitate the transport of sodium chloride from the loop of Henle in the kidney, as a result of which water is absorbed in the distal convoluted tubule and less urine is produced. Frusemide, a loop diuretic, blocks the action of enzymes in the loop of Henle and thus less sodium chloride is transported across the membrane. Without sodium chloride uptake, water is not absorbed from the distal tubules and diuresis is increased.

Cell membrane transport

Movement of electrolytes across cell membranes enables function of many kinds of cells, including nerves and muscle fibres. Electrolytes pass through ion channels in cell membranes, but channel opening can be blocked or enhanced by different drugs that bind at, or near, the ion channels.

For example, drugs used to control cardiac arrhythmias do so by blocking ion channels and the flow of electrolytes across the myocardial cell membranes. This reduces the rate of depolarisation. Lidocaine, given intravenously, will block ion channels and the fast influx of sodium ions into cells, slowing down depolarisation and thus the disorganised, rapid contracting of the myocardium in ventricular tachycardia.

Anti-metabolites and cytotoxic agents

These drugs kill specific cells. Anti-metabolites are similar in chemical nature to nutrient molecules, which cells need in order to function. However, they do not provide the cell with the nutrient it requires and so although the chemical is absorbed by the cells, the lack of the nutrient results in the cell's death. An example of this is the drug methotrexate, which resembles folic acid without which rapidly dividing cells will die. Methotrexate is often given in conjunction with Folinic acid to counteract the anti-folate action of Methotrexate on normal cells.

Cytotoxic drugs affect cell function and survival by interfering with DNA or RNA structure or synthesis, inhibiting protein synthesis and cell division. Numerous cytotoxic drugs used in cancer chemotherapy have these effects, including cyclophosphamide, cisplatin or paclitaxel (Taxol). Antibiotics and antiviral drugs similarly interfere with bacterial or viral cells' ability to live and reproduce.

PHARMACOKINETICS

The way a drug is handled in the body will affect how the drug is used and prescribed in respect of the dose, frequency, duration of treatment and possibly the route of administration. In some circumstances the route of administration is governed by other factors, such as the patient's state of health or the preparation the drug is available in. For example, antibiotics may be given intravenously initially to achieve a sufficiently high plasma level, after which oral administration will maintain the serum levels at the required level until the course is complete. Bioavailability of a drug refers to the proportion of the original amount given which is available in the circulation; it is dependent on many factors.

The dose

The amount given will affect the amount available in the bloodstream, by whatever route the drug is given. There is a balance to be struck between achieving an adequate level of serum concentration in order to achieve a response, and having a toxic level of the drug. This is known as the therapeutic index or window (Hopkins & Kelly 1999).

The route

The bioavailability and time a drug takes to act depend significantly on the route by which it is administered. Drugs given intravenously have 100% bioavailability on administration and act rapidly. This is in contrast to those administered orally whose bioavailablity is lower and is affected by their absorption from the gastrointestinal tract and metabolism in the liver before they reach the remainder of the systemic circulation.

Distribution

Once in the bloodstream, which compartments and tissues the drug travels to affects the serum levels and the site of action of the drug. Some drugs remain in the bloodstream only. Within the circulation some molecules of the drug bind to plasma proteins. The quantity of the drug which is bound is no longer available for therapeutic use, only the remaining amount which is free in the plasma is active. Some drugs diffuse out of the circulation to the extracellular or interstitial fluid. Other drugs enter the cells or are even found to concentrate intracellularly, as opposed to being evenly distributed between all the compartments (intravascular, extracellular and intracellular). The further the drug diffuses through the body, the lower the available concentration of a drug at any given site of action.

For example, 1 mg of a drug which remains in the intravascular compartment has a higher concentration there than 1 mg of a drug which diffuses through all compartments. Drugs given intravenously affect the peripheral tissues only after all the organs with a high blood flow have been perfused with blood containing the drug.

Elimination

The duration of a drug's action is affected by the speed at which it is metabolised or excreted. Prescribing is guided by the drug's half-life, that is the time taken for serum concentration to decrease by a half or 50%. Serum levels of a drug are also influenced by how the body metabolises or excretes it. Drugs which are rapidly excreted may need to be given frequently or by continuous infusion, whilst those excreted slowly need to be given less often. Drugs which are excreted slowly, such as digoxin, may need to be given with a large loading dose followed by smaller doses to achieve and maintain a steady bioavailability.

Metabolism

Liver enzymes break down or inactivate chemicals, including many drugs and alcohol. If the liver is damaged (as in patients with cirrhosis or hepatitis) or its circulation is impaired (as in patients with cardiac failure), its function may be slowed and its ability to deal with drugs impaired. Some drugs affect liver enzymes, either enhancing or decreasing their action, which can have a knock-on effect in their metabolism of other drugs. Changes in liver function or prescribing certain drugs will influence the prescribing of other drugs, as well as their doses and frequency of administration.

Excretion

The kidneys excrete many drugs or their breakdown products and so renal function will affect serum levels of certain drugs. Patients with renal failure, and the elderly, often require reduced doses of these drugs, such as gentamicin. Other drugs or their breakdown products are excreted in bile and then via the gastrointestinal tract; rarely they may be excreted from the lungs (Trounce & Gould 2000).

Drug interactions

When patients are prescribed several drugs there is a danger that the drugs may interact, with serious and adverse consequences. Interactions can take a physical, chemical or therapeutic form. Physical interactions can be seen in the form of precipitate forming or colour change. Chemical changes arise from alterations in the molecular structures of the compounds involved and may be visible with precipitate or colour changes, or may not be visible at all. Therapeutic incompatibilities are those which occur when two drugs interact to inhibit the effect of one or both of the drugs. These interactions can happen at a number of sites and is a significant potential problem for patients having intravenous therapy. Drugs may interact in the container or tubing they are administered in, in the blood, at the site of action of the drugs or at the sites of elimination of the drugs.

Reactions occur between different drugs (chemicals) based on their different pH, or differently charged ions combining (for example, calcium and phosphate to form calcium phosphate precipitate), or molecules combining to inactivate one or both of the compounds involved. Precipitate causes problems either by blocking the venous device, damaging veins or capillaries and causing phlebitis, or by introducing emboli into the circulation. If any obvious change occurs to a solution with one or more drugs in it, *it must not be administered to the patient* and a pharmacist's advice must be sought. Even drugs that appear to be of the same group or type may still not be compatible and this should always be checked, never assumed. If no information can be found about the compatibility of two drugs then they *should not be given together*.

Some drugs interact with the container through which they are administered to reduce their efficacy. For example, nitrates interact with PVC, as does insulin, both drugs leaching out into the plastic, reducing the amount of drug being given to the patient. For this reason, infusions and tubing through which drugs are infused should be changed every 24 hours.

Ideally, intravenous drugs should never be given at the same time through the same venous access device unless the device is a multi-lumen central venous catheter and different lumens are used. Sometimes this is unavoidable, especially in critically ill patients, and in these cases it must be established that the drugs are compatible before administering them. When several drugs are given through a venous access device it must be thoroughly flushed with 0.9% sodium chloride before, between and after administration of each drug to avoid mixing of drugs and to ensure complete delivery of the dose into the patient's circulation.

Other influencing factors

Age and weight

Both these factors influence the doses of drugs a patient should be prescribed. The larger a person is, the lower the concentration a standard dose of a drug will achieve and thus the less intense its effect. Doses can be calculated either on weight alone, or more accurately using height and weight to achieve the patient's surface area. Then drug doses are calculated per square metre of body surface area using a nomogram (Weinstein 2001).

Babies and children require small amounts of drugs due to their small size, their fluid and electrolyte distribution and the degree to which the organs involved in metabolism and excretion have developed. Thus doses are usually calculated using age to weight or age to skin surface ratios.

The elderly also require different doses of many drugs to avoid toxicity. A safe and therapeutic dose for a person at 35 years of age could cause toxic reactions for the same person at 70. This is due to the deterioration of metabolism and excretion, as the liver and kidneys have reduced blood flow and enzyme function is diminished.

Nutrition

Patients who are malnourished will respond differently to a drug from someone who is well nourished. This is related to loss of body mass and a reduction of enzyme activity due to diminished protein intake.

Race and genetics

Genetic and cultural differences, including those which affect diet and lifestyle, influence drug metabolism. This can be on an individual level as well as a population level.

Illness

Illnesses affecting organs involved in drug distribution (cardiovascular system and the gut), metabolism (liver) or excretion (kidneys and gut) will affect either receptor/ligand binding and/or drug elimination from the body. This has implications for the particular drugs used for a patient and the doses prescribed.

Drug stability

Drugs are usually produced by manufacturers in a stable form for storage and are dispensed with information leaflets or data sheets about their reconstitution, administration and storage. Drugs can become unstable with toxic by-products, or inactive when irreversible reactions change their properties from their original form. For these reasons manufacturers' guidance about the drug must be adhered to. The factors that affect the stability of drugs are described in Table 6.1.

Table 6.1 Factors affecting drug stability

Factor	Effect
pH	A drug's composition after reconstitution with the recommended diluent, is designed to result in a pH at which the drug remains stable. Mixing drugs with the wrong diluent, in the wrong sequence, with the wrong volume of diluent or infusion fluid or another drug could affect the pH of the solution and result in the drug losing its stability and either becoming inactive, or developing a precipitate (phenytoin added to 5% dextrose will have a low pH and develop a precipitate).
Diluent	As described above, using the correct volume of the correct diluent is vital to maintain the stability of a drug. 5% dextrose solution is acidic and, depending on the drug, may be required (sodium nitroprusside) or actively avoided (vancomycin) when reconstituting or administering a drug depending on its properties (erythromycin to be diluted with 5% dextrose makes an acidic solution – a buffer must be added to neutralise it. Alternatively it can be diluted in 0.9% sodium chloride without requiring a buffer).

Table 6.1 *Continued*

Factor	Effect
Other drugs	Reactions with other drugs will affect a drug's chemical stability and could be harmful for the patient (ampicillin and gentamycin are *not* compatible). Giving drugs together intravenously is to be avoided, and compatibility must be checked whenever it is unavoidable.
Time	Drugs will decompose in time and the state the drug is in affects its stability over time (cyclosporin must be infused within six hours once mixed for infusion). A shelf life of several years may change to a few hours once a drug is reconstituted for administration (ampicillin is only stable for one hour when reconstituted with 5% dextrose). Manufacturers' guidelines must be followed and expiry dates carefully checked prior to administration of any drug.
Temperature	Heat provides energy for chemical reactions and some drugs will not be stable at relatively low temperatures. Stability at particular temperatures often changes once a drug is reconstituted, and those that can be stored at room temperature are not stable at room temperature once reconstituted. Alternatively those stored in a fridge may only be stable at room temperature for a short time. Always store drugs at the recommended temperature.
Light	Light also provides energy for some chemical reactions. Some drugs are unstable in light, either after reconstitution, or at any time. Light will cause them to break down into either non-therapeutic products or toxic ones. These drugs need to be protected from light as stated by the manufacturer. This may mean avoiding direct sunlight (frusemide), covering an infusion bag with a dark cover (vitamins, e.g. Multibionta), or using a light-sensitive administration set to prevent any exposure of the drug to light (sodium nitroprusside).

MONITORING DRUG LEVELS AND EFFECTS

In order that the therapeutic index (level of drug obtaining the desired response without provoking toxic reactions) is achieved in a patient's therapy, it may be necessary to measure the serum level of the drug in question at regular intervals and then have the dose adjusted as indicated by the results. Patients prescribed intravenous gentamicin or digoxin may require monitoring of their serum levels and dose adjustment to ensure a therapeutic level is achieved without toxicity. The timing of blood sampling for monitoring serum drug levels depends on the drug in question, and it is important to establish the correct time to take blood in relation to the last or next dose, so that an accurate measurement is obtained. If the patient has a CVC in situ it is preferable not to draw blood from the catheter for serum levels if the drug has been given through the same device. If this is unavoidable, it should be indicated on the sample request form. The catheter lumen must be flushed well with 0.9% sodium chloride solution after administration of the drug, and before drawing the blood, to remove traces of the drug which could affect the sample level.

Different timings of intravenous drug administration

Intravenous drugs can be given in one of three ways, as regards the time of administration.

(1) A bolus dose.
(2) An intermittent infusion.
(3) Continuous infusion.

The decision as to which method to choose is based on the circumstances, the required serum level of the drug to be achieved balanced against reducing the risk of a reaction, and toxic effects of giving a drug too quickly.

Bolus dose

When a peak level is required in a matter of minutes a drug may be given by a bolus dose – that is, direct injection from a

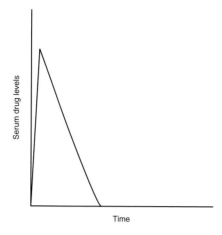

Fig. 6.1 Serum level of a drug over time when given as a single bolus dose

syringe into a venous access device (or directly into a vein, though this is less common in in-patient settings or long-term therapy): see Fig. 6.1. Bolus injections should usually be given over several minutes to avoid 'speed-shock' or 'red man syndrome' (Chapter 4 p 115).

When a drug that needs to be administered rapidly (such as adrenaline/epinephrine in an emergency cardiac arrest situation) it can be given as an 'intravenous push'. It is rapidly administered as fast as possible and followed with a flush of 0.9% sodium chloride or 5% dextrose to ensure it is delivered into the circulation. When administering drugs as a bolus, great care must be taken to ensure the venous access device in use is correctly situated and is patent and that there is no phlebitis in the vein in question. Administering an intravenous bolus dose of a drug can lead to phlebitis if given too rapidly, may cause devastating tissue damage if infiltration or extravasation of the drug occurs, and can cause a rapid anaphylactic reaction.

Administering a drug by a bolus dose is feasible only when it is possible to inject the volume that the drug is delivered in, over the time required and stated by the drug manufacturer. Drugs needing dilution in volumes greater than those easily administered in a syringe will need to be given in intermittent infusions. Details of how to administer a drug in a bolus dose can be found in Chapter 4 (p 116).

Intermittent infusion

When a drug is administered as an intermittent infusion, a larger volume can be given over a longer period of time and achieve intermittent peak serum levels (see Fig. 6.2). Some drugs, such as potassium chloride, vancomycin or erythromycin, have to be given in this way because their toxic nature and need for dilution preclude their administration intravenously as a bolus dose. This method of administration still achieves peak levels of a drug, though not as rapidly. It is useful when a peak level is therapeutically desirable but the drug needs dilution to avoid toxic reactions. It can also be used when a drug is incompatible with a fluid being given in a continuous infusion and needs to be given intermittently whilst the fluid infusion is temporarily stopped. Details of how to administer a drug in an intermittent infusion can be found in Chapter 4 (p 120).

Continuous infusion

A continuous infusion of a drug is achieved using a syringe pump or infusion bag to achieve a steady serum level of the drug (see Fig. 6.3). This is important when the half-life of a drug is very short (minutes) or a constant therapeutic dose is required. Patients receiving continuous infusions will require monitoring during the infusion to ascertain the effect of the drug and detect any adverse effects early. Continuous infusions may be titrated (adjusted) according to the patient's response to the drug, such as insulin or glyceryl trinitrate

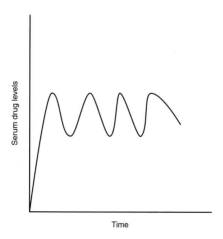

Fig. 6.2 Serum level of a drug over time when given as intermittent infusions

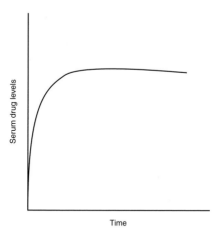

Fig. 6.3 Serum level of a drug over time when given as a continuous infusion

Table 6.2 The advantages, disadvantages and implications of giving drugs intravenously

Advantages	Disadvantages	Implications
Rapid action	Increased risk of toxicity and reaction especially with rapid administration	Drugs need to be given at an appropriate rate and dilution for their action and potential toxicity.
100% bioavailablity on administration	Infection is a significant risk with potentially lethal consequences	Asepsis is mandatory in all aspects of intravenous therapy and venous access device management.
Can achieve a constant blood level with a continuous infusion	Phlebitis and thrombophlebitis	Drugs must be appropriately diluted and given at the recommended rate.
		Appropriate devices must be used for their purpose and the type of vein to be cannulated.
		Devices must be removed from peripheral veins after 72 hours and earlier if signs of phlebitis are visible or there is any difficulty infusing through them.
		CVADs and PICCs should not be used if thrombophlebitis is suspected, and expert help sought.

Enables administration of drugs not available in other preparations	Risk of emboli from thrombosis, precipitates or particles in the infusion	Thrombosed veins must not be used – see above. Drugs should not be given in combination to avoid interaction. Drugs must be properly reconstituted with the appropriate type and volume of diluent. They must be administered using the correct size of needles and dilution to avoid the infusion of particles.
Smaller doses are required to achieve a therapeutic effect	Risk of air embolism particularly with central venous catheters	Positioning the patient head down (preferably) or at least lying flat for insertion and removal of central venous catheters is vital to avoid air embolus. All infusions must be carefully prepared and infused to avoid air embolus. When using non-collapsible containers with air inlets, infusions must be stopped before the container empties completely.
Avoids using the oral/enteral route	Increased risk of severe anaphylaxis	All staff involved in administering intravenous therapy must be competent in recognising anaphylaxis. They must be conversant with local policy on anaphylaxis management and be able to

Table 6.2 *Continued*

Advantages	Disadvantages	Implications
Avoids the first pass effect on drugs absorbed from the gut, passing through the liver	Once administered the drug cannot be removed and reversal is difficult	take emergency measures to manage a patient suffering such a reaction. Practitioners administering intravenous therapy must be competent and familiar with the drugs prescribed in their area of practice so as to minimise inappropriate drug administration and reactions.
	Red blood cells are easily damaged by hypertonic or hypotonic solutions	Drugs must be reconstituted according to manufacturer's recommendations. Non-isotonic solutions must be administered slowly and continuously as prescribed.
	Extravasation of cytotoxic drugs can cause tissue necrosis	Vascular access devices must be checked for patency prior to giving cytotoxic drugs. These drugs must be administered by specially trained and experienced practitioners

Circulatory overload can be induced with excessive infusion of large volumes of fluid

Incompatibility of drugs or their diluents can result in reduced efficacy or damaging effects for the patient.

Intravenous infusions must be administered as prescribed and the patient's condition monitored throughout.

Elderly or critically ill patients must be closely monitored for signs of circulatory overload.

Drugs should not be given intravenously through the same device at the same time. If this is unavoidable compatibility must be checked beforehand.

Drugs must be reconstituted according to manufacturer's recommendations.

Drugs which undergo an obvious change (forming precipitate or colour change) must not be given, and a pharmacist's advice must be sought.

infusions. Details of how to administer a drug in a continuous infusion can be found in Chapter 4 (p 126).

THE IMPLICATIONS OF USING
THE INTRAVENOUS ROUTE

Giving drugs intravenously is undoubtedly potentially hazardous without an understanding of the implications of doing so. Table 6.2 lists the benefits and disadvantages, as well as the implications of using the intravenous route for drug administration.

DRUG CALCULATIONS

It is important that all practitioners involved in drug administration can calculate drug doses, volumes and infusion rates accurately and quickly. As described in Chapter 1, each practitioner is accountable for decisions they make in practice, including checking (or deciding not to check) drugs they are administering and the volumes and rates they are administering the drugs in (Hutton 1998). Where a practitioner feels that they wish to verify a calculation with someone else, both should undertake the calculation and then cross-check their answers, rather than one person relying on the other's working. There is always a risk of deferring to another's answer when it is perceived that that other person must be right because of their status, authority or experience. This is not necessarily the case and both practitioners must agree the answer together, having both undertaken the calculation separately first and compared workings. Woodrow (1998) suggests tips for doing drug calculations:

- use calculators, information and other aids;
- take time, avoid interruptions and recheck answers;
- do calculations safely, not to show off mental arithmetic skills;
- if unsure of the calculation or answer, *do not give the drug*, get help;
- answers that look wrong usually are wrong.

Box 6.1 Standard international units of weight and volume

Units of weight:
  1 kilogram (kg)   = 1000 grams (g)
  1 gram (g)   = 1000 milligrams (mg)
  1 milligram (mg)   = 1000 micrograms (mcg or μg)
  1 microgram (mcg or μg)   = 1000 nanograms (ng)

NB Micrograms and nanograms should preferably be written in full to avoid confusion.

Units of volume:
  1 litre (l)   = 1000 millilitres (ml)
  1 millilitre (ml)   = 1000 microlitres (mcl or μl)

NB Microlitres should preferably be written in full to avoid confusion.

It can be helpful to estimate the rough amount to be given and compare this with the answer obtained (Hutton 1998).

Standard international units (SI units)

All drug doses and volumes are counted in SI units. When calculations are done, the same unit of measurement needs to be used in a calculation, so knowledge of units is essential (see Box 6.1). This is because in any calculation, the same units must be used to achieve the right answer. If a drug is dispensed in vials containing 1 gram and the dose prescribed is 500 mg, milligrams must be used in the calculation, and thus the 1 g will change to 1000 mg.

When calculating using SI units it is useful to revise multiplication and division using decimal points to simplify the arithmetic (see Box 6.2).

Formulae

There are a few simple formulae that will help to calculate concentrations and volumes easily (see Boxes 6.3 and 6.4). It is important to remember always to use the *same units* in any

---

Box 6.2 Multiplication, division and decimal points

Multiplication and decimal points:

To multiply by	Move the decimal point
10	1 place right
100	2 places right
1000	3 places right

Division and decimal points:

To divide by	Move the decimal point
10	1 place left
100	2 places left
1000	3 places left

Box 6.3 Formulae for calculating concentrations, doses and volumes

To calculate doses, concentrations and volumes:

$$\frac{\text{What you want}}{\text{What you've got}} \times \text{Volume you've got} = \text{Volume required}$$

or

$$\frac{\text{Dose prescribed}}{\text{Dose available}} \times \text{Volume of solution} = \text{Volume required}$$

Remember always to use the same units and change units if necessary.

For example: Gentamicin prescription, 120 mg, IV, 12 hourly.

$$\frac{120 \text{ mg}}{160 \text{ mg}} \times 2 \text{ ml} = 1.5 \text{ ml}$$

$$\frac{12}{16} \times 2$$

$$= \frac{3}{4} \times 2$$

$$= \frac{6}{4} = \frac{3}{2} = 1.5 \text{ ml of gentamicin } 80 \text{ mg/ml } 2 \text{ ml ampoule}$$

> **Box 6.4** Formulae for calculating infusion rates
>
> To calculate infusion rates in millilitres per hour:
>
> $$\frac{\text{Volume prescribed (ml)}}{\text{Hours of infusion time}} = \text{ml/hour}$$
>
> To calculate infusion rates in drops per minute:
>
> $$\frac{\text{Volume prescribed (ml)}}{\text{Hours of infusion time}} \times \frac{\text{Drops per ml of giving set}}{60 \text{ (minutes per hour)}}$$
> $$= \text{drops/minute}$$
>
> Remember always to use the same units and change units if necessary. This applies to minutes and hours as well as volumes and weights.
>
> For example: 1 litre 0.9% sodium chloride prescribed over eight hours
>
> (a) how many millilitres per hour and
> (b) how many drops per minute through a standard administration set?
>
> (a) $\dfrac{1 \text{ litre}}{8 \text{ hours}} = \text{ml/hour} = \dfrac{1000 \text{ ml}}{8 \text{ hours}} = 125 \text{ ml/hr}$
>
> (b) $\dfrac{1000}{8} \times \dfrac{20}{60} = \text{drops/min}$
>
> $\qquad 125 \times \dfrac{1}{3} = \dfrac{125}{3} = 41.7 \text{ drops/min}$
>
> $\qquad\qquad\qquad = 42 \text{ drops/minute}$

calculation; change the units if necessary so that they are the same.

When calculating infusion rates for administration sets, the drops per millilitre value is always printed on a specific administration set's wrapper:

- blood administration sets = 15 drops per millilitre;
- standard administration sets = 20 drops per millilitre;
- metriset or dosifix burette administration set = 60 drops per millilitre.

> **Box 6.5** Formula for calculating infusion rates for drugs prescribed per kilogram of a patient's weight
>
> $$\text{ml/hour} = \frac{\text{microgram/kg/min} \times \text{Patient's weight kg} \times 60 \text{ (min/hour)}}{\text{Solution concentration in micrograms per ml}}$$
>
> or
>
> micrograms/kg/minute
>
> $$= \frac{\text{ml/hour} \times \text{Concentration in mcg/ml}}{\text{Weight in kg} \times 60 \text{ (mins/hour)}}$$
>
> Remember to keep units the same.
>
> For example: a prescription of dopamine in a solution of 1.6 mg/ml is to run at 2 micrograms/kg/min and the patient weighs 60 kg. What is the hourly rate of the infusion?
>
> $$\text{ml/hr} = \frac{2 \text{ (micrograms/kg/min)} \times 60 \text{ (kg)} \times 60 \text{ (min)}}{1.6 \text{ (mg/ml)} \times 1000 \text{ (to correct to micrograms)}}$$
>
> $$\text{ml/hr} = \frac{7200}{1600} = \frac{72}{16} = \frac{18}{4} = 4.5 \text{ ml/hr}$$

When an infusion rate is to be calculated for a drug prescribed per kilogram of the patient's weight, such as inotropes, two further formulae are needed; see Box 6.5.

Percentages

Some solutions are expressed as percentages rather than mg/ml; crystalloid solutions are an obvious example (5% dextrose or 0.9% sodium chloride). A percentage value expresses the weight of the drug in grams per 100 ml of water, or percentage weight in volume (%w/v).

5% dextrose = 5 g in 100 ml

or

5000 mg in 100 ml

It is important to be able to calculate the dose in mg or g of a drug a patient receives from a percentage solution.

Ratios

Other solutions are expressed as a ratio. This means the number of grams of the drug dissolved in a given volume of the solution. A solution of 1:1000 is one where 1 g of the drug is dissolved in 1000 ml.

For example, adrenaline (epinephrine) is dispensed in 1:1000 solution. To give 0.5 mg of 1:1000 solution to a patient experiencing anaphylaxis:

$1\,g$ is in $1000\,ml = 1000\,mg$ in $1000\,ml = 1\,mg/ml$

$\dfrac{0.5\,mg}{1\,ml} \times 1\,ml = 0.5\,ml$ would be administered.

TEST INTRAVENOUS DRUG DOSE CALCULATIONS

These questions are intended to mirror the kinds of drug calculations that commonly need to be undertaken in practice. Answers with workings are at the end of the chapter. Try working them out without the answers and then check against the answers provided. All working should be written down and checked. This is what should happen in practice where two practitioners each do the calculation, with workings shown, and then compare answers. Both must be satisfied that they agree with the final answer and how it was achieved, regardless of their respective roles or expertise.

(1) Convert the following into micrograms:
    (a) 0.5 mg   (b) 0.25 mg   (c) 0.0625 mg

(2) Convert the following into milligrams:
    (a) 300 micrograms   (b) 75 micrograms
    (c) 187.5 micrograms

(3) Convert the following into grams:
    (a) 34 mg   (b) 518 mg   (c) 1785 mg

(4) You have a prescription for 10 mg of pethidine for Mr Jones. The injection strength in the controlled drugs cabinet is 50 mg/ml. What volume would you give?

(5) Mrs Barrett has been prescribed 0.4 mg buprenorphine. The available stock is 300 micrograms/ml. What volume do you give Mrs Barrett?

(6) The strength of digoxin injection in the drugs cupboard is 500 micrograms in 2 ml. What volume do you need for a dose of:
(a) 0.125 mg?   (b) 375 micrograms?

(7) A patient is prescribed phenytoin, IV, 300 mg at night. The injection you have in the drugs cupboard is 250 mg in 5 ml. What volume will you draw up?

(8) A patient with septicaemia is prescribed benzylpenicillin, metronidazole and gentamicin for broad-spectrum therapy before the causative organism has been identified.
(a) The benzylpenicillin is prescribed as 1.8 g, IV, six hourly. You have vials of 600 mg, each of which needs to be reconstituted with 5 ml of sterile water for injection. At this strength/dilution, how many ml will be needed to give the 1.8 g dose?
(b) If this volume is added to 100 ml of 0.9% sodium chloride to be infused over 30 minutes, what is the infusion rate in ml/hour?
(c) Metronidazole 500 mg, IV, every eight hours was prescribed. This is to be given over 30 minutes. You have 500 mg pre-prepared in a 100 ml infusion bag. Using a standard administration set, what will the infusion rate be in drops per minute?
(d) The gentamicin is prescribed as 350 mg, IV, daily for two days. The ampoules available contain

80 mg in 2 ml. What volume is needed for this dose?

(9) Calculate the amount of the drug (in milligrams) in the volumes specified for the following solutions:
   (a) 10 ml of 10% dextrose
   (b) 20 ml of 0.2% lidocaine
   (c) 5 ml of 20% mannitol
   (d) 100 ml of 0.1% glyceryl trinitrate

(10) Mr Humphries is prescribed a dose of 4800 mg of calcium gluconate 10%, IV, over 24 hours. Calculate the flow rate in ml/hour.

(11) Mr Singh is prescribed 40 000 units of heparin in 0.9% sodium chloride, IV, over 24 hours. The vial of heparin is 25 000 units/ml. The infusion is prescribed to run at 1 ml/hour.
   (a) What volume of heparin should be drawn up?
   (b) How much 0.9% sodium chloride should the heparin be mixed in to infuse to 40 000 units over 24 hours (at 1 ml/hour)?

(12) Miss Jacobs needs 0.5 mg adrenaline (epinephrine). The ward stock is 1:1000.
   (a) What volume needs to be drawn up?
   (b) If Miss Jacobs then requires 1 mg, and the only solution available is 1:10 000, what volume would be needed?

(13) Mrs Marley is prescribed dobutamine 500 mg in 250 ml 5% dextrose to infuse at 10 micrograms/kg/minute. Mrs Marley's weight is estimated at 50 kg.
   (a) Calculate the flow rate in ml/hour.
   (b) Calculate the flow rate in drops per minute (assuming a standard administrations set with 20 drops/ml is to be used).

INFORMATION RESOURCES

In current practice, it is impossible to commit to memory all the information available about issues related to practice. In respect of pharmacology alone, memorising every drug that may be encountered routinely in one area of clinical practice would be challenging. For this reason, it is far more important to have a working knowledge of commonly encountered practice issues and pharmacology, and to know where to obtain reliable information and advice about those aspects less frequently encountered. For intravenous drug administration there are many resources available to practitioners to facilitate safe and effective intravenous therapy for patients. Most of these should be available or accessible locally in the clinical area or institution where care is delivered or planned (for patients in the community). Other resources may require more investigation to retrieve from other institutions, libraries or drug companies. Table 6.3 contains a suggested list of resources to support intravenous drug administration and those practitioners learning and involved in intravenous therapy.

Table 6.3 Information resources for practitioners giving IV therapy

Resource	Comment
Data sheets with drugs	For comprehensive information about storing, reconstituting, and administering a drug, its prescribing, incompatibilities and interactions.
ABPI data sheet compendium *British National Formulary*	A collection of data sheets for many drugs currently available. Appendix of intravenous additives lists drugs given intravenously, which method they can be given by and suitable diluents.
Ward pharmacist	For information and advice about specific drugs, interactions or pharmacological advice on incidents relating to drug administration.
On-call pharmacist	As above out of working hours.
Drug information unit	Comprehensive information about all drugs from specialist centres.
Local policies and guidelines	Information about drug administration and drugs the employer has approved for practitioners to administer. Guidelines about intravenous therapy and its administration by employees in general and specific circumstances. Policies need to be adhered to by practitioners for reasons of vicarious liability (see Chapter 1).
Hospital/Trust intranet	Many Trusts have local and national policies, guidelines and other information to support evidence-based practice available on their local computer network.
Internet	Specialist sites may have information about national policy, drugs, practice issues, educational information, equipment and more. Information on the internet may not be evidence- or research-based and should be used thoughtfully and selectively.
More experienced colleagues	People of the same and other professions who work in the same area or in adjacent ones, usually have experience or know where to get advice.

Remember to change units so they are the same:
$0.125 \, \text{mg} \times 1000 = 125$ micrograms

$$\frac{125}{500} \times 2 \, \text{ml} = 0.5 \, \text{ml}$$

(b) **1.5 ml**

$$\frac{\text{want}}{\text{got}} \times \text{vol} = \text{volume required}$$

$$\frac{375}{500} \times 2 \, \text{ml} = 1.5 \, \text{ml}$$

(7) **6 ml**

$$\frac{\text{want}}{\text{got}} \times \text{vol} = \text{volume required}$$

$$\frac{300}{250} \times 5 \, \text{ml} = 6 \, \text{ml}$$

(8) (a) **15 ml**

$$\frac{\text{want}}{\text{got}} \times \text{vol} = \text{volume required}$$

Remember to change units so they are the same:
$1.8 \, \text{g} \times 1000 = 1800 \, \text{mg}$

$$\frac{1800}{600} \times 5 \, \text{ml} = 15 \, \text{ml}$$

(b) **230 ml/hr**

$$\frac{\text{volume prescribed}}{\text{hours of infusion time}} = \text{ml/hour}$$

Volume = 100 ml + 15 ml of benzylpenicillin = 115 ml

$$\frac{115}{0.5} = 230 \, \text{ml/hour}$$

NB Some manufacturers' infusion bags contain 5–10% excess volume, others contain the exact volume. The important thing is to infuse the whole amount whether or not the volume of the drug is added to the total volume in the bag.

(c) **67 drops per minute**

$$\frac{\text{volume prescribed}}{60 \text{ mins (1 hour)}} \times \frac{\text{drops/min}}{\text{hours of infusion time}}$$

$$\frac{100}{60} \times \frac{20}{0.5} = 66.6, \text{ round up to 67 drops/min}$$

(d) **8.75 ml**

$$\frac{\text{want}}{\text{got}} \times \text{vol} = \text{volume required}$$

$$\frac{350}{80} \times 2 \text{ ml} = 8.75 \text{ ml}$$

(9) (a) **1 g or 1000 mg**

10% solution = 10 g in 100 ml

$$1 \text{ ml} = \frac{10 \text{ g}}{100 \text{ ml}} = 0.1 \text{ g/ml}$$

10 ml = 0.1 g × 10 ml = 1 g

Multiply by 1000 to get mg: 0.1 × 1000 = 100 mg/ml
10 ml = 100 mg × 10 ml = 1000 mg

(b) **40 mg**

0.2% solution = 0.2 g in 100 ml

Multiply by 1000 to get mg: 0.2 × 1000 = 200 mg

$$1 \text{ ml} = \frac{200 \text{ mg}}{100 \text{ ml}} = 2 \text{ mg/ml}$$

20 ml = 2 mg × 20 ml = 40 mg

(c) **1 g or 1000 mg**

20% solution = 20 g in 100 ml

$$1\,ml = \frac{20\,g}{100\,ml} = 0.2\,g/ml$$

5 ml = 0.2 g × 5 ml = 1 g

Multiply by 1000 to get mg: 0.2 × 1000 = 200 mg/ml
5 ml = 200 mg × 5 ml = 1000 mg

(d) **100 mg**

0.1% solution = 0.1 g in 100 ml

Multiply by 1000 to get mg: 0.1 g × 1000 = 100 mg

$$1\,ml = \frac{100\,mg}{100\,ml} = 1\,mg/ml$$

100 ml = 1 mg × 100 ml = 100 mg

(10) **2 ml/hour**

10% solution = 10 g in 100 ml

Remember to change units so they are the same:
10 g in 100 ml × 1000 = 10 000 mg in 100 ml

$$1\,ml = \frac{10\,000\,mg}{100} = 100\,mg/ml$$

$$\frac{want}{got} \times vol = volume\ required$$

$$\frac{4800}{100} \times 1\,ml = 48\,ml\ in\ 24\ hours$$

$$\frac{volume\ prescribed}{hours\ of\ infusion} = ml/hour$$

$$\frac{48}{24} = 2\,\text{ml/hour}$$

(11) (a) **1.6 ml**

$$\frac{\text{want}}{\text{got}} \times \text{vol} = \text{volume required}$$

$$\frac{40\,000}{25\,000} \times 1\,\text{ml} = 1.6\,\text{ml}$$

(b) **22.4 ml**

To run @ 1 ml/hour over 24 hours, need 24 ml
24 ml − 1.6 ml = 22.4 ml of 0.9% sodium chloride
solution

(12) (a) **0.5 ml**

1 : 1000 = 1 g in 1000 ml = 1000 mg in 1000 ml = 1 mg/ml

$$\frac{\text{want}}{\text{got}} \times \text{vol} = \text{volume required}$$

Remember to change units so they are the same:
1 mg in 1 ml × 1000 = 1000 micrograms/ml

$$\frac{500}{1000} \times 1\,\text{ml} = 0.5\,\text{ml}$$

(b) **10 ml**

1 : 10 000 = 1 g in 10 000 ml = 1000 mg in 10 000 ml =
0.1 mg/ml

$$\frac{\text{want}}{\text{got}} \times \text{vol} = \text{volume required}$$

Remember to change units so they are the same:
0.1 mg in 1 ml × 1000 = 100 micrograms/ml
1 mg × 1000 = 1000 micrograms

$$\frac{1000}{100} \times 1\,\text{ml} = 10\,\text{ml}$$

(13) (a) **15 ml/hour**

Dobutamine solution of 500 mg in 250 ml

$$\frac{500}{250} = 2\,\text{mg/ml}$$

Remember to change units so they are the same (micrograms prescribed):

$2\,\text{mg} \times 1000 = 2000$ micrograms/ml

$$\frac{\text{micrograms/kg/min} \times \text{patient's weight (kg)} \times 60\,(\text{mins/hour})}{\text{micrograms per ml of dobutamine solution}}$$
$$= \text{ml/hour}$$

$$\frac{10 \times 50 \times 60}{2000} = 15\,\text{ml/hour}$$

(b) **5 drops per minute**

$$\frac{\text{vol. prescribed (ml)}}{\text{hours of infusion time}} \times \frac{\text{drops/ml of set}}{60\,(\text{mins/hour})}$$

$$\frac{15}{1} \times \frac{20}{60} = \frac{300}{60} = 5\,\text{dpm}$$

REFERENCES

Hopkins, S.J. & Kelly, J.C. (1999) *Drugs and Pharmacology for Nurses* 13th edn. Churchill Livingstone, Edinburgh.

Hutton, M. (1998) Numeracy skills for intravenous calculations. *Nursing Standard* **12**(34), 49–56.

Trounce, J. & Gould, D. (2000) *Clinical Pharmacology for Nurses* 16th edn. Churchill Livingstone, Edinburgh.

Weinstein, S.M. (2001) *Plumer's Principles and Practice of Intravenous Therapy* 7th edn. Lippincott, Philadelphia.

Woodrow, P. (1998) Numeracy skills. *Nursing Standard* **12**(30), 48–55.

ADDITIONAL TEXTS

Coben, D. & Atere-Roberts, E. (1996) *Carefree Calculations for Health Care Students*. Macmillan, London.

Gatford, J.D. & Anderson, R.E. (1998) *Nursing Calculations* 5th edn. Churchill Livingstone, Edinburgh.

Shulman, R., Drayon, S., Harries, M., Hoare, D. & Badcott, S. (1998) *UCL Hospitals Injectable Drug Administration Guide*. Blackwell Science, Oxford.

WEBSITES

British National Formulary
http://www.bnf.org

Medicines and Healthcare products Regulatory Agency – information and standards relating to medicines and medical equipment used in England
http://www.mhra.gov.uk

Index